DISABILITY AND TH

Disability and Theatre: A Practical Manual for Inclusion in the Arts is a step-by-step manual on how to create inclusive theatre, including how and where to find actors, how to publicize productions, run rehearsals, act intricate scenes like fights and battles, work with unions, contracts, and agents, and deal with technical issues. This practical information was born from the author's seventeen years of running the first inclusive theatre company in New York City, and is applicable to any performance level: children's theatre, community theatre, regional theatre, touring companies, Broadway and academic theatre. This book features anecdotal case studies that emphasize problem solving, real-world application and realistic action plans. A comprehensive Companion Website provides additional guidelines and hands-on worksheets.

Stephanie Barton-Farcas is the Artistic Director of Nicu's Spoon Theater Company. Founded in 2001, it is the first company in NYC history to be fully inclusive (age, gender, color, religion, disability, nationality). She is also the co-founder of the Disability Cinema Coalition. She recently directed *Richard III* with a disabled cast except for the title role, and her company Nicu's Spoon is the subject of the documentary *Two and Twenty Troubles* which follows the production of *The Cherry Orchard* and four of the disabled actors in it. She has been profiled in *The NY Times*, *Variety*, *American Theatre Magazine* and *Playbill* as a director and advocate. As a writer she has been published in *Backstage*, *Howlround* and many other disability or theatre publications as well as lecturing and teaching at SAG-AFTRA, AEA, and many film and theatre industry associations and colleges (Columbia, NYU) in the US and in Europe (CEU in Hungary, University of Riga, University of Kiev, Royal Conservatoire Scotland among others) about inclusion in the arts.

Dedicated to my mother, and every mother that has given their child a gift of a diverse and inclusive world, not an 'us vs. them' world.

Dedicated to my child, and every child with an artists heart. Go and change the world and never give up.

CONTENTS

FIGURES

NOTES ON CONTRIBUTORS

Sean Williams is a playwright/actor/producer living in New York. He has written for *Slate*, *The Huffington Post* and *The New Yorker*, and has a memoir coming out in 2018. He's been the executive producer of Gideon Productions for the last sixteen years, where he has produced shows that have consistently earned rave reviews (including critic's picks in *The New York Times*, *Village Voice*, *Time Out New York* and *The New York Post*). He's produced shows at 59E59, The Lucille Lortel, 45 Bleeker, The Harry de Jur, Soho Playhouse and The Gym at Judson. He has acted in more than sixty plays.

Bryce Alexander (Artistic Director of Naples Players in Naples, Florida) was Artistic Director of Phamaly Theatre Company from 2009 to late 2016. Two of Bryce's major accomplishments include leading Phamaly on its first international tour to Osaka, Japan, where he facilitated a series of community workshops to promote inclusion and the effective application of disability theory in both western and traditional Japanese art forms; and helping to lead a regional 'Sensory Summit' in Denver, CO, to provide arts and cultural organizations with the knowledge and tools they need to produce their own sensory-friendly programs – an initiative that garnered Phamaly two Denver Mayor's Awards for Arts & Culture. Bryce is a member of the Society of American Fight Directors and an associate member of the Stage Directors and Choreographers Society, and his work from major regional theatres to various small community venues around the US has given him a well-rounded perspective on the significance and importance of accessibility in the arts.

Christine Bruno is an actor, director, acting coach and disability advocate, and received her MFA in acting and directing from the New School in New York. She is a lifetime member of the Actors Studio and has worked across all mediums. A proud union member, Christine is Chair of the New York SAG-AFTRA Performers with Disabilities Committee and serves on the SAG-AFTRA National Performers with Disabilities and the Actors' Equity EEOC Committees. As Disability Advocate for Inclusion in the Arts, she has represented the organization at symposiums, film and theatre festivals, forums, panels, resource events and television and radio outlets across the US and internationally. Her selected theatre, film and television credits include *The Maids* (adaptation by Jose Rivera, INTAR), *The Glass Menagerie* (Fulton Theatre), *The Good Daughter* (NJ Rep), *The Ugly Girl* and *Raspberry* (musicals, UK), *Screw You, Jimmy Choo!* (UK and Australia), *Law & Order, iCreep, Flatbush Luck* and *This is Where We Live.*

Deborah Emmy Nowinski is the founder of Dionysus Inclusive Theatre Company in Texas (www.dionysustheatre.net). She is a director, educator, speaker and playwright. Deborah also leads workshops and seminars for Texas educators on the benefit of inclusion theatre. She served on the City of Houston Commission for People with Disabilities where she chaired the Emergency Preparedness Committee. Deborah has received the City of Houston's Mayor's Advocate of the Year, American Blind Council Vision Award and the City of Houston Commission for People with Disabilities Care Award.

Stephanie Barton-Farcas is the founder and Artistic Director of Nicu's Spoon Theater Company (www.spoontheater.org), based in New York City and Hawaii. She is also the co-founder of the Disability Cinema Coalition and sits on the board of Identity Theater Company. Nicu's Spoon has been a WNYC's 'Salute the Arts (STAR)' Initiative winner, an *Off Off Broadway Review* (OOBR) award winner, a multiple New York Innovative Theatre Award (NYITA) winner, the Thom Fluellen Award winner for service to New York City as well as winner of the

Snapple/NYC Mayor's Office Best People to Work For Award and many more. The company has been spotlighted in *Playbill*, *The New York Times* and many others, and was also the subject of the documentary *Two and Twenty Troubles*. Stephanie herself is a mother, writer, speaker, actress, director and producer and has been nominated for the Encore Award from the Arts and Business Council of New York, is an Alliance of New York State Arts Organizations 'Advancing Cultural Development' Award nominee, a NYITA winner, an OOBR award winner, a runner up in the L'Oréal Humanitarian Award as well as Reviewfix naming her as one of Top 10 Off or Off-Off Broadway Professionals in New York City. She teaches privately for acting, auditioning and accent work on takelessons.com and is at work on a second book, *Acting & Auditioning for the 21st Century*.

Joan Lipkin divides her time between New York City and St Louis, where she is the founder and Artistic Director of That Uppity Theatre Company (www.uppityco.com). She is also the co-founder of The DisAbility Project, one of the oldest ensembles in the US to produce original work about disability who are also included in the permanent collection of the Missouri History Museum. In addition to people with disabilities, she has also devised work with numerous populations including women with cancer, LGBTQIA youth and adults and their families, seniors, adolescent girls, college students, women who have been sexually trafficked and exploited, people in recovery from substance abuse, communities of faith and youth at risk. An award-winning playwright, director, educator and producer, Joan has received the Association for Theatre in Higher Education Award for Leadership in Community-Based Theatre and Civic Engagement, a Visionary Award, the Arts Innovator of the Year and the Ethical Humanist of the Year, among many others. Her writing is widely anthologized.

ACKNOWLEDGMENTS

To Julie Campbell and Natalie Blair, my co-founders from day one. And for my mother, Mihai, and Sam who keep me sane. To the Spoonies – all 2,500 plus of you around the world. I love you all.

To Henry Holden, John Belluso, Ike Shambelan, Joe Genera and Nicu. All gone too soon.

Special thanks to contributors and inspirations Bryce Alexander (Bryce was Artistic Director of Phamaly Theatre Company until late 2016 and now is in Naples, Florida making art there), Christine Bruno, Talleri Macrae, Lawrence Carter-Long, Deborah Nowinski, Joan Lipkin and her assistant Becky Galambos, Sean Williams and Brad Rothbart. Deborah has written a book already, but every one of you should too!

PREFACE

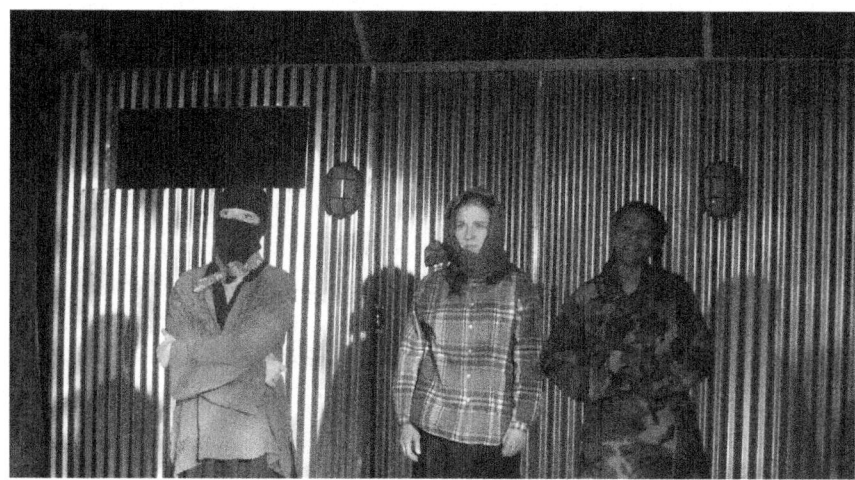

Figure 0.1   *Displaced* by S. Barton-Farcas, Natalie Blair, Gina Daniels, Julie Cambell and Jo Yang. Directed by S. Barton-Farcas, *Nicu's Spoon*, 2001. L to R Natalie Blair, Julie Campbell and Gina Daniels. (Photograph courtesy of Nicu's Spoon Theater Company.)

I am not a disability scholar, although I do know quite a bit about the history of disability and the study of it. Disability history is our shared history as a country whether we acknowledge it or not, as we will all be disabled one day. I am not an activist, although I am an advocate for full inclusion in all things, free expression of art and thought and am a believer in a new theory of accessibility which demands full accessibility for all people in all places at all times. This capitalizes on the growing universal design movement, which seeks to create buildings not specifically accessible for the disabled, but which encompass the spirit of being completely accessible for all people equally. It is a matter of equity, not equality. Equity is inherent fairness in all ways, equality means everyone gets the same thing. Not everyone needs the same things, however, which is why equity is what we need, not equality. Imagine a world in which every person can enter, move around in and access every room in every single building.

I have been told I am an idealist in my goals to have fully inclusive theatre and full equity as a true functional and ongoing aspect of our artistic society. Yet, I am not an idealist, I am in fact a realist. As cultures shift and politics and paradigms change, it seems the artists who survive the change are the realists. I just do not think many theatre makers, universities, regional theatres, board members or funders (whether they be state, federal, local or independent foundations) are being attentive to the reality we have in this increasingly inclusive and global world.

My company, Nicu's Spoon Theater, fosters inclusion and disability culture and artists with disabilities, staff, boards, designers, composers and playwrights in theatre. This is distinguished from 'disability theatre' in that my company's work refers to making art that defies the social norms and includes disabled people, whether in themes, ideas, performance or the creation of the artwork, rather than works focusing on disability as the central theme (although we have done disability theatre works on occasion). We practice what I term 'cross-disability casting' which is the casting of artists with disabilities, but frequently not in a role with the disability they possess. Our inclusive casting (which also includes colors, genders and ages) and the word inclusion can also refer to any work we make that is made as a political or social act geared toward shaping a new theatrical community which then enhances disability culture, or in our case inclusion culture.

The term 'disability' in actuality usually refers to about six distinct types of disability: visual impairment, hearing impairment, mobility impairment, cognitive or developmental impairment, degenerative diseases which impair the body, and then the umbrella term 'general impairments' which is used to encompass every other disability. In the USA, because of diet and health care we have eliminated disabilities that are common in other parts of the world (gout, elephantiasis and cleft palate are only a few examples) and what we have not eliminated we can quickly do plastic surgery on. We eradicate. However, this does not mean we can eradicate the larger picture and the much larger politically and socially aware disability population as a whole.

My company, now in its seventeenth season, is by no means the be-all and end-all of theatre. We have been a small to medium group in the very large pond that is New York City. We became known because we fought against convention, did not accept the status quo and came prepared to argue our point and fight, if needed, for the vision of inclusive theatre that we had. We spoke out, hosted panels, invested energy in community and disability groups and activities, experimented onstage with language, bodies, text and kinesiology, wrote articles, cast entirely in new and risky ways and produced endlessly. We tried and tried and sometimes failed. We tried to use our failures as the gateways into creation, investment and risk-taking on stage. We then picked ourselves up and continued to try and then, to teach. We became very well known in that small pond. I am certain this book may provoke strong reactions as we expand outward and put forth our own theories and experiences (our work goes into a global setting in our seventeenth season, with a multi-country project, GLOBE), as I have already been taken to task during the very writing of this book by one company director for not wording their case study, which I had written for them, in 'person-first language' (PFL).

Although I do not practice person-first language and prefer identity-first language (IFL) which names someone as autistic much as someone would be called gay or Jewish (my belief being that saying disabled person or autistic person validates them as that person, that individual, as a person of worth as a disabled or autistic person), many do prefer PFL. Thus, I immediately apologized to this company director as this is only one of many polarizing issues within the vast disability community. If you yourself do not know what person-first or identity-first language is then read on, this book is for you.

By the very nature of inclusive theatre and the push towards 'reality-based' casting, inclusion is political in essence and has many social ramifications. The very makeup of the sheer diversity of types of disabilities within the disabled spectrum lends itself to the fact that oftentimes it is the social, political and activist connections that bond these differing disabled bodies together. If then artists with disabilities are to be cast in leading roles on stage and in film, then society must adjust accordingly and provide for them in all ways, in all places and spaces at all times, and that is not how it currently works. When an actor with cerebral palsy (CP) is employed or cast in a role, it advances all artists who happen to have CP, however it does nothing for blind artists, those who are little people, those on the autism spectrum and so forth. Again it is the diversity of the 'disability story' that can make it seemingly work against itself.

The study of disability culture is a study then of not just the blind, or those with multiple sclerosis (MS) or traumatic brain injuries (TBIs) but a study of the entirety of those who do not match the physical and societal status quo. In reading disability history, and in fact in creating it, do we then choose the history of the blind artist, the little person, the girl with autism, the boy with a spinal degeneration? There are so many roots in the ground that make up the tree of disability history, culture and studies. That is why we must look at the tree as a whole.

Universal design encompasses this concept and indeed the concepts behind much inclusive theatre. Many workplaces, schools, theatres and offices continue to not be accessible (and any time the word access is mentioned one should also automatically attach the word 'egress' to it – entry *and* exit – it may seem the same thing to you until you are in a wheelchair which does not enter *and* exit unless you have space to turn around) even though there are laws in place to force them to be accessible. There are even places with what Blogger Mike Ervin calls 'coattail' access. These are places where the accessibility is purely accidental, such as shopping malls or grocery stores with automatic doors or ramps which were built in the back of buildings to allow for the removal of the large garbage cans or containers, but which made the building 'coattail' accessible. This access was never planned, but it now exists and literally is a way of slipping (or rolling) in the back door. The very act of slipping in the back door and practicing inclusive theatre or disability theatre is, in itself, a political and social statement.

I have written about inclusive theatre many times both online and in print as well as having spoken and lectured about it and hosted panels on it for the past seventeen years. I was lucky enough to attend a conference in 2005 hosted by The Public Theater in New York City where I met many of those whose shoulders we all stand on. Simi Linton, the bawdy and beloved author and activist, and John Belluso, the intensely brilliant playwright (I admit to a horrible crush on John) were only a few I met then and what I remember is how clearly they all spoke. How clearly we all need to speak to each other to be understood. Thus, I prefer to speak in the plainest terms possible at all times in this book so that practitioners, academics, teachers and artists alike can understand and use my points and ideas. Clarity encourages understanding. The artists and designers and staff I have worked with over the past seventeen years and the disabilities they have represented have schooled me well on being clear with them as opposed to pedantic, verbose, politically or socially motivated and overly academic. So, this tome will invariably be in plain language terms, as will the case studies presented by the various practitioners. The case studies are likewise presented in three clear parts, History, Plan and Outcome (outcomes are the bulk of Chapter 16) and in simple non-academic English. This book set out to be one thing and that was, and is, practical thus plain English is needed.

In early 2001 I co-founded, with two other actresses, the first fully inclusive theatre company in New York history (and still continue to be stunned nobody else was doing this inclusive work at all then in New York City, the apex of new works and ideas). I had been lucky enough to have been raised to appreciate people for who they were with no regard to disability, color, sexuality or nationality. I remember as a young actor watching my very heavy and adored acting teacher, Diana Bellamy, perform as Amanda Wingfield in *The Glass Menagerie*, by Tennessee Williams and feeling my brain expand. She was the finest Amanda I have ever seen before or since, and I have seen many. Why couldn't a very heavy actress play the role? Or a black one? Or one with one leg? Or one who was deaf? Being exposed to disability in my own family as well as colors and nationalities imbued me with an open mind. It helps if you have one as well.

It seemed, in 2001, almost every New York City theatre company was spouting the word 'inclusive' yet very few had people of color performing, disabled writers writing, women on their board, older company members and so forth. Exhausted with the lip service, and exhausted by those telling me to produce works about white men and women because audiences would like that, we founded Nicu's Spoon. There is a story behind the name of the company.

I worked with abandoned kids in Romania in the 1990s and the most amazing one was Nicu, who was five. Nicu was in diapers and did not walk, talk or feed himself. They told me he was deaf and mute and 'retarded' and hopeless. Nicu had spent five years on his back in a crib. They told me he was a lost cause and could not be worked with. I got angry at that and said "I'll take him." Six months later he did all those things. He and I fought some big, bad battles together to get him there – to get him to choose life. And in the process he changed my life. Though he was mentally and physically challenged, Nicu viewed the world with wonder. He spent hours bouncing sunlight off of a spoon. When he began to eat solid food at the age of five, his spoon was everything to him. Nicu's spoon became the symbol for us for all the impossible things that were suddenly possible. Things like walking, talking, thinking and living. He was HIV positive and we lost him five years later in 1996. Nicu's life was about quality, not quantity, about life's impossibles becoming possible. The company thus echoes those things and works with and for people who may be told "it is impossible." Because it is possible, it is all possible.

Over the past seventeen years I have produced over forty full length plays (every one with artists with disabilities in them) off and off-off Broadway and directed over half of them as well as produced over forty-five workshops and staged readings of new plays (twenty-two of which featured disabled roles and/or were written by disabled playwrights). We have worked with well over 2,500 actors, writers, designers, composers, directors, crew, staff and board and artists of all kinds in that time. They delight in calling themselves Spoonies. My company, Nicu's Spoon, actively recruits and works with every disability imaginable as well as every age, gender, color, sexual identity, religion, language and nationality.

I define the artists I speak about in this book as anyone (actors, writers, composers, designers, staff and crew) who creates art. I also use, except in two cases, full and real names of the artists I speak about in my own company case studies. Why? So that you will search them out and hire them, of course. Disabled artists need employment. They have huge value in artistic society and their value is not dependent upon them becoming the norm, but in showing us and teaching us an entirely new 'norm.'

There is a long, frustrating and fascinating history in disability studies, about the history of the struggle for the Americans with Disabilities Act (ADA) signed in 1990, or the UK's Disability Discrimination Act (1995), the history of the language we use or do not use in order to label varying disabilities, the ongoing struggle and history in regard to equal training and employment and some of all of that we will touch on in this book, but this book is not about those things. This book is, quite simply, about how to recruit, cast, staff, produce and create professional quality fully inclusive theatre with an emphasis on working with artists with disabilities. This book proposes a new theory of accessibility, postulates new ways to problem solve and encourages new modes of thinking to replace archaic ones.

This book is about how to invite disabled people and artists to be on your boards, direct your plays, be your dramaturgs, crew, playwrights, designers and actors. This book is about how to do it right, like true working professionals do, with humor and love, how to work directly with all kinds of artists while ignoring the myths about it. This book is a confirmation that your needs, the project's needs and the disabled artists' needs cannot be approached separately. There is always a balance, a yin/yang in this kind of theatre. This is the theatre of the future, an all inclusive future. No matter what political or social restrictions may come in the arts, this is the theatre of the future. This book is about how to implement it all one step at a time and how to come out of it with a great artistic experience for everyone including your audience. Of course a great audience experience translates into a healthy box office, reviews and artistic satisfaction.

However, none of this can continue to work without the growing systemic change in how we recruit, educate, create and open up jobs for artists with disabilities. It is not enough for a university campus to be ADA compliant if they do not actively recruit, encourage and grow new artists, writers and thinkers. This doesn't even count the disabled stage managers, facility managers, the non-creative staff of the theatrical and academic world. The system itself must change. Theatres and universities must change. This book then gives everyone some of the pathways where they can stop wondering about working with disabilities in theatre and thus, take action.

I am often asked if I am disabled myself. I choose not to answer and here is why. If I am disabled then the story becomes about this brave disabled woman who makes theatre, and that is not the story I want to tell. If I am not disabled then the story becomes about this good Samaritan who helps those less fortunate, and that is not the story I want to tell. I choose not to answer because the story I want to tell is about the disabled artists, writers, designers and thinkers and the creation of new performance styles, ways to problem solve and creatively perform. That is the story we need to focus on in this country.

Theatre should be innovative, fresh, shocking, creating active debate and thought. Rarely should theatre be safe and boring. Even if you do a revival of a well-known play it can still be filled with excitement and newness and passion. If not, then why do it? Why do "Meh, it was ok…" theatre? That is the death of art and theatre. If theatre does not reflect our true global society, in all colors, abilities, genders, ages, lifestyles, religions and nationalities, then it does not reflect society at all. Not truly. It is just another play written by a white, male playwright (and yes, I know many great white, male playwrights, but I am making a point) directed by the same and starring the same. Boring with a capital B.

That 'same-ness' is not my daily reality, not the world I see on the streets of New York, not on the streets of Europe, not in this global and increasingly high-tech world. Theatres that have their heads stuck in the 1930s where, "Gee, we're all white fellas and we're going to do a show!" are sadly and horribly out of touch with twenty-first century reality. The über wealthy patrons and the foundations that support these theatres are out of touch as well, and it both saddens and angers me. Do not get me started thinking about opera houses funded by the wealthy, although they are already rolling in funds and wasting $5,000 for a gold gilded pair of shoes for their soprano, or the National Endowment for the Arts (NEA) and its active funding primarily of the same companies over and over again who do not always do anything new and creative to earn it. For younger and newer companies in the US, the NEA application process is so complicated and convoluted that it alone often stops them from applying for funds. This is an artistic pity, as these smaller companies are the ones actively writing the new plays, producing new artists and exploring new theatrical boundaries.

We need as artists, directors, writers, companies and academic institutions to not only produce more reality reflective, socially challenging theatre, but we also need to bring more educators, funders and donors to it and by bringing them to it we then educate them. Too often theatre companies and individual artists may take the role of educator upon themselves when they should not have to, teaching prospective funders what working with artists with disabilities really means. Academic and arts training programs need to open up nationally and both actively recruit and accept more disabled artists into their ranks as well. If training programs do not do this they will rapidly find themselves falling behind as the disability community grows in social and political power. In the twenty-first century the disability community in the US is rapidly becoming more vocal, more political, writing books, sitting on panels, snagging those university jobs, doing public speaking and becoming a major political force for cultural change.

Sharon Barnartt is professor and chairperson of the Department of Sociology at Gallaudet University and has argued that usage of the concept of 'culture' does not adhere to the usual anthropological definitions. Rather, she suggests that the concept of collective consciousness much better describes what is occurring in the disability community in the twenty-first century than does the term 'disability culture.' While a culture functions to maintain the social order, a collective consciousness impels the actions which comprise social and political movements. This is what is happening in the disabled communities across the US this very day. Those who make art are on the front lines of reflecting to the rest of the world what the world really looks like (when you pay attention to it) so we ourselves must pay attention to it.

You, universities, training programs, academics and academic recruiters, audition boards, theatre companies, regional theatres, you must begin to broaden your creative horizon, begin to look at colors, ages, genders, disabilities, nationalities. There is literally a rainbow of different artists waiting for you to work with them in this world. Do not miss it because you are stuck in a rut or afraid to start, or your board doesn't get it. There is no 'Pride' group which represents the disabled community. Yet. However, it is coming, in one way or another. The world is changing fast, you need to take risks, make big moves and keep up or you will find yourself, your company, your university wondering where your students and audiences went.

1

WHY THIS BOOK?

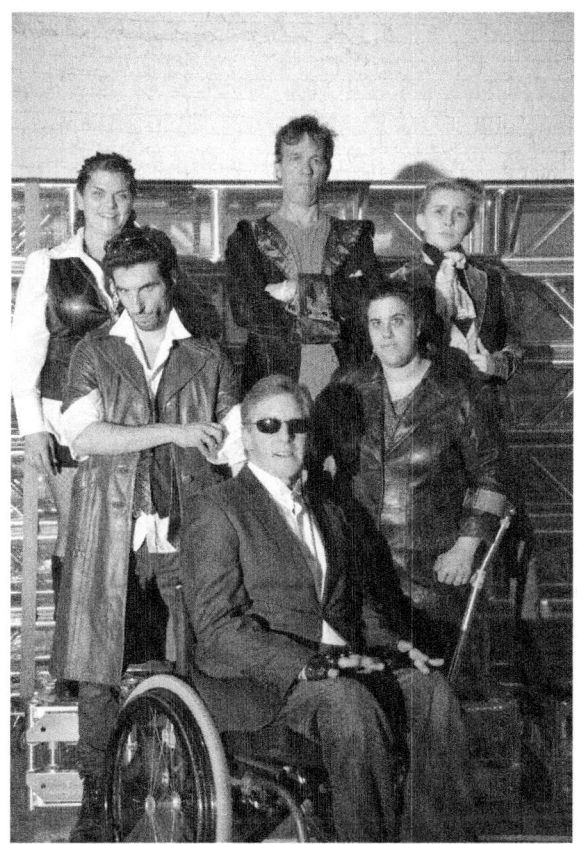

Figure 1.1 *Richard III* by William Shakespeare, 2015. Our production had every cast member except Richard III, and thus the society of the play, as disabled. L to R back row, Jessica Levesque as Clarence, Guy Ventoliere as Richard III, Estelle Olivia as Prince Edward, center L to R Perri Yaniv as Clarence (yep 2 Clarences!), Stephanie Gould as Norfolk and Joe Genera as Catesby. (Photograph courtesy of Nicu's Spoon Theater Company.)

Why this book you may ask? Because there is not another 'process' book about this anywhere. There is no professional or academic manual about how to recruit, cast, rehearse, train and perform with a hugely diverse cast and with an emphasis on disabled artists. There is no other book that has cobbled together best practices from theatres working in this area. The de-mystifying and de-stigmatizing of this work must also be undertaken and this process must be disseminated to a wider audience, especially in the US and other countries where 'normal' is the apex of being and any deviation from it continues to be stigmatized and politicized. The investment in these communities must be emphasized and increased.

The 2016 election has polarized the US, however for those of us in the arts it only increases our ongoing and vital mandate that we practice active inclusion of all genders, sexual orientations, colors, races, religions and nationalities and disabilities. Art crosses political lines and emphasizes compassion and fairness. Art also energizes and inspires those who are marginalized to carry on as human beings. Art creates new platforms from which to create, speak and galvanize new audiences. This is part and parcel of our responsibility as arts makers and leaders. Far too often even those artists and teachers who work in this area are either too swamped to share their lessons and best practices or too worried about competition for funding or politics to share their 'secrets' to working. This has to change if this work is to grow and deepen. This has to change if we are to grow as artists and as a country.

This book will be anecdotal in many sections as it is the true human experience that needs to be shared to begin this de-mystifying process. Frequently in a historical, political or social context it has been the reluctance to view disabled people (and all the other marginalized groups I have worked with) as human that has propagated the mistreatment of them. Thus, anecdotal information and real-world experience casts us all in a real light and reveals artists with disabilities as the human beings they have always been. It serves as a reminder of the process we need to undertake. It's not that academic English has no place in this, it is simply that it can be used as a distancing mechanism, in a way becoming a dialect of privilege, and that we do not want in this book.

A new way to think about accessibility has begun to happen in both the theatre and the academic community, as well as socially and politically. A new accessible theory which stops being a theory, stops non-dissemination of process and technique, stops encouraging ableism (the discrimination in favor of able-bodied people), encourages time and investment and thus goes into practice. While racist or sexist comments are often intentionally discriminatory, ableism is ingrained in our culture and people do not realize they're propagating it. It's often not driven by hatred or hostility, like discrimination towards a different race or gender, but comes from misguided compassion and societally reinforced pity and habit.

This book is by no means a manifesto, however, by virtue of the political climate in the US in the past, disability issues have always been set in a political context. By virtue of the societal baggage inherent in working with the disabled the subject matter has taken on, certainly, emotional, historical, vocabulary, political and personal undertones as well. So, all of these political, emotional and personal issues will be addressed in this book. There may be detractors who say, "These issues have nothing to do with staging for disability theatre or inclusion theatre." However, it is my belief that these are in fact at the very foundation of this ongoing work. These undertones need to begin to be emphasized and taught in more academic settings as well.

What this book is: this is a detailed and user-friendly how-to manual essentially from start to finish. How to find, audition, rehearse, tech, perform, design, PR and market, run and close a professional full-length show with a variety of performers and staff and crew who are disabled involved. All colors, genders, ages and disabilities. This book mostly, out of necessity, focuses on the artists with disabilities, but all of these standards are applicable to all marginalized groups. My company has, over the seventeen years we have produced, worked with artists with Human Immunodeficiency Virus/Acquired Immune Deficiency Syndrome (HIV/AIDS), cerebral palsy (CP), blindness, deafness, multiple sclerosis (MS), epilepsy, many artists on the autism spectrum, amputees, alcoholics, stutterers, those who have had polio and spina bifida, little people, burn victims, those with cancer, artists with a spectrum of birth defects and/or degenerative diseases, traumatic brain injuries (TBIs), sensory integration disorder, muscular dystrophy, developmental disorders, stroke, bipolar disorders, manic depressives, severe asthmatics, spinal cord injuries and many more. You can work together with them too.

Thus, this book is not a heavily footnoted discourse on the lack of foundation in previous theories written about in this field. There are not many major theories in this field, although I would encourage reading in disability studies in general. This book is not an uplifting saga of disabled folks that will soon be a movie of the week. The artists and practitioners do not need that type of yadda-yadda. Disabled artists (as well as older, gay, transgendered, immigrant and so forth) want and need equal training, work and support and creative problem solving as artists, and really don't we all want that? Disabled artists and activists are now working daily to ensure they get respect, jobs and work. The international disabled community understands that they must take media coverage, social activism and politics into their own hands. They do not need pity or placation, just solid formal training, work and support.

When approached from a practitioner point of view there is nothing more difficult about making art with artists with disabilities than with anyone else. It is past time to get pity and old assumptions about the needs or the costs or the 'problems' of working with disabled artists set straight. Those academics or casting directors out there with the outdated assumptions often are the ones hiring local artists and running theatres and they have to get on board with the reality of it all. It is their job to remove obstacles to creating art and give the community what it needs. Obstacles do not only refer to the physical. Some of those obstacles may in fact be other people and the societal acceptance of certain behaviors the non-disabled think nothing of. For one simple example, far too many non-disabled people use handicapped bathroom stalls and take up space in crowded elevators, paying no attention to those with disabilities who do not have any other options, without a second thought. Parking in handicapped parking spaces to quickly run into a store has also become ingrained in our society as something to do, 'real quick'.

While these actions may not (or may) be meant meanly, they are hard and fast evidence of the way non-disabled privilege still manifests in our society. What manifests in our society is what continues to be represented in casting, educational training, employment and vocabulary. These are key areas where all obstacles must be removed.

Significant obstacles continue to exist for individuals with disabilities who want to pursue careers in the arts. Things like lack of access to solid, appropriate, professional training and education in the arts, limited exposure to updated information and resources about the range of career opportunities as artists, arts technicians or arts administrators, as well as lack of formal training, recruitment or hiring opportunities at all (especially in the technical, management and design fields). Couple these issues with lack of familial support, lack of role models, lack of hiring in academic settings, lack of support from recruiters, fear of losing disability benefits, lack of support from counselors and art programs and it seems impossible (and we haven't even mentioned getting cast). The worst thing is the constant stereotyped rejection of disability content in the arts, or disabled artists in general, as essentially maudlin and not up to professional standards.

Many theatre companies and producers continue to have fears about assimilating artists with disabilities into the larger arts community, believing it will cause restrictions on funding or loss of box office revenue and audiences (actually I have found the reverse to be true), worrying about endless transportation and accommodation needs, and loss of their own funds due to benefits planning for artists with disabilities. These fears are greatly unfounded and stem from lack of information and completely archaic notions. As long as you have all the realistic information you need and look at it seriously those concerns melt away.

The problem is that most universities, regional theatres or theatre production companies do not want to look at this seriously. They do not really want those concerns to melt away. It is easier to not think about it. But the world catches up with you and audiences are much more savvy nowadays. In truth it is no more time consuming working with a disabled artist than it is dealing with an actor who has memorization problems and no more expensive than dealing with an actor who has a hard commute into New York City from New Jersey for rehearsals.

For those artists with disabilities who get the training and become artists and technicians and designers, the top three areas identified by them as their priorities to really advance their careers are their professional development in professional (paying) settings, funding and financial costs and strategies on how to work and yet keep their disability benefits (and this last issue is one they grapple with alone, usually not one that impacts their employers). It is up to us, as the practitioners who can hire them to address these issues with them and use this deep well of human resources in our collective art.

Let us be frank as well about the organizations not wanting to actively work with disabled artists because they fear the artists won't be good enough, the productions won't be good enough or that they will have to ask their audience to applaud substandard work out of pity. This fear usually comes from those very people who do not make an effort to create any educational or casting opportunities for these same artists to get training to be good enough to applaud for. It becomes a repetitive cycle of non change. These are the organizations most in need of change. Enough of this. These are all outdated ideologies and just not true.

This book not only takes you step-by-step through the entire production process, but comes with a variety of short case studies or an action plan at the end of most chapters. Most of the case studies illustrate creative problem solving and a successful outcome, but not all. Perhaps the most important case studies are where the problems were only partially solved or not solved at all, for then we learn what does not work. The case studies do illustrate the most important aspect though, trying. Trying to work and problem solve and create. Just getting started, that is what is important.

Who is this book then for? Practitioners and human resource folks first and foremost, drama therapists, board members, community theatres, regional and local theatres, any theatre company of any size and makeup, directing and producing students in college, theatre and stage management students, academics and their classes, architects and theatre planners, fundraisers, grant writers, stage management students, social scientists, scholars in the humanities, disability rights advocates, creative writers and others concerned with the issues of people with disabilities, college recruiters and educators, casting directors, disabled advocates and activists and artists of all kinds.

It is time to get serious about training and creating work with artists with disabilities, with one in five Americans having a disability and one in six eligible voters being disabled (and with each battle we fight overseas that increases as our veterans return home) and globally around 550 million disabled people. My company has, over the past seventeen years, staged original works, company-generated works, classics, Shakespeare, musicals, Pulitzer Prize winners, children's shows, plays by disabled and non-disabled playwrights and has done it all with an enormous spectrum of disabled artists. Let go of your fears and read this book. It will give you needed information and some starting places so that you and/or your organization can move forward creatively. If you ignore artists with disabilities, then you ignore twenty percent of your audience base and twenty percent of a wealth of talent. Get more information so you can do the work.

Case Study 1: A Seizure Onstage, Nicu's Spoon Theater, New York City

History

So, what do I mean by having all the information? In order to produce theatre and work with disabled artists you must know certain things about them. Sometimes they may not tell you those things and you find out the hard way.

Our company, Nicu's Spoon, was founded in 2001 and was producing its second show ever in 2002 in a theatre in midtown Manhattan, an *extremely* well-known play which had had heavy audience attendance. Expectations were very high for the play itself and for this production. We had a cast of sixteen made up of five nationalities and nearly one-quarter of our cast was disabled, though at least one had a 'hidden disability.' Some common hidden or 'invisible' disabilities include TBI, epilepsy, HIV/AIDS, post-traumatic stress disorder (PTSD), attention deficit hyperactivity disorder (ADHD), psychiatric disorders and many others that have no immediate outward signs yet are permanent disabilities. Being in our second year of production I had some passing experience with hidden disabilities in my life background and at that time the term 'hidden disabilities' was only starting to be talked about as new disabilities were added to it.

One of the young actors in a fairly major role had a hidden disability, he was epileptic, and only one person in the cast knew about it. That one person was not me nor the production staff. The play proceeded that night as usual and I was aware that this actor's divorced parents were in the audience that night, causing him some stress. He had not been eating or sleeping well as a result. He was an extremely talented young man, and also very skinny and a bit physically delicate. Nearly ten minutes into the play mid-sentence his eyes rolled up into his head and he slammed to the ground in a grand mal epileptic seizure. The actors onstage froze, the audience froze, the production staff and technicians froze and the play screeched to a stop.

Plan

What would you do next? What we did is in the back of this book, but you work this out. You have a full audience in midtown Manhattan, who have paid to see this well-known, Pulitzer Prize winning play and they have seen only ten minutes of it. You have fifteen fellow actors who are now traumatized and angered by this ongoing seizure, you have no doctor on staff, and none of the production staff, or you, the producer, knew he had epilepsy, and so on. What do you do? How do you save face, save the show, save the actor and still keep your profits?

Now, in working with artists with disabilities (any artists, really) you should always have them disclose *anything* to you that can interrupt the play (seizures, aversion to strobe lights, allergy to fog machines or wool, etc.) but some may not. A terrific way to handle hidden disabilities is to talk early to the full cast and explain what hidden disability means at a cast meeting, the first read-through is appropriate, and simply request that anyone with anything to share should let you know privately.

There is an 'intimacy of disability' when working with disabled artists, an intimacy because you as director or producer are privy to knowledge about an artist's body (and their emotions) and how it functions in a way you are usually not privy to with a non-disabled artist. This circle of intimacy is a very special place to work with an artist and is as important, if not more so, as the practical work you do with them. Many times I have talked with artists who were not born with a disability, but became disabled later in life. I always tell them that they are still an artist, but now they are a different artist. They still have a body, but now it is just a different body. I can only say this and be heard (and being heard is the important part) if I am already in a circle of intimacy with them.

They must be assured their privacy is respected, but you must also know any and all issues that can drastically affect a show. Them disclosing to you and only you (and the stage manager) is enough, but the show should never be put at risk because you as the producer or director do not have all the information you need. This show and that seizure taught us that lesson.

See Chapter 16 for further details of this case study.

2

WHAT IS INCLUSION?

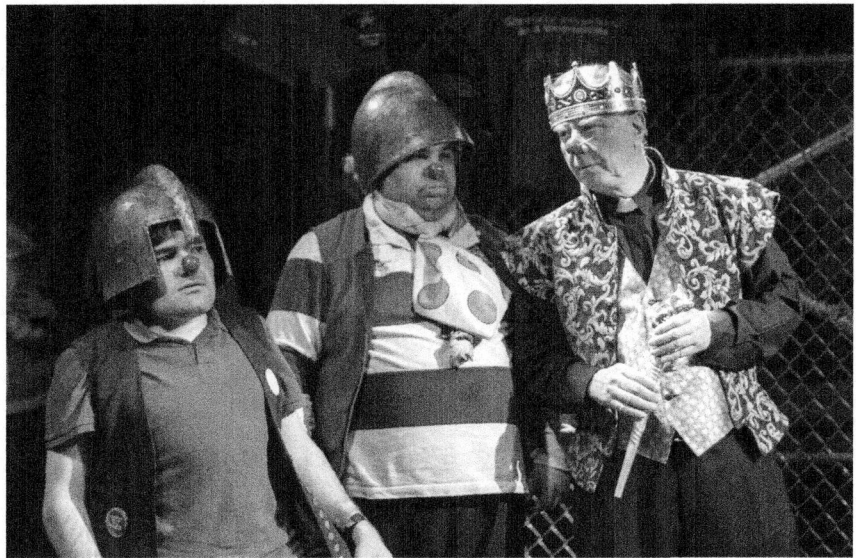

Figure 2.1   *Red Noses* by Peter Barnes, 2015, Nicu's Spoon Company. L to R
Alexander Nero as LeGrue, Nick Linnehan as Bembo and James Harter
as Father Flote. (Photograph courtesy of Rhesa Storms.)

'The state of being taken in, as part of a whole.' Inclusion, for my
company, is a vast range of things; the intersections of politics
and aesthetics and identity and empowerment. We believe the
stage can serve as a place of freedom and rebirth for people with
disabilities. What would that idea then look like? What indeed?
What are the possibilities when you embrace the full possibilities
of intersectionality of inclusion? Inclusion and disability theatre are
terms that are inherently deviations from the social, cultural and

political normative. The term inclusion is thrown around a lot these days but most theatre companies aren't quite sure what it is and some just do not care. Academics, and even funders and corporations, often do not understand it as well and must be educated. For me it is the involvement of *all* marginalized groups. All colors, races, religions, nationalities, ages, genders, LGBTQIA (lesbian, gay, bisexual, transgendered and questioning, intersex and asexual), disabled and women. This is again different than 'disability theatre,' which is theatre groups who work specifically with one or more segments of the disabled population. We do that as well, and have worked in tandem with many companies that do that. We embrace the reality that *every* body and form on a stage impacts how the bodies of the audience feel. We work with professional performance standards with all disabilities and all colors, genders, ages, nationalities. We understand that disability is a social category as much as gender, color or religion. Now, in our seventeenth season we are a conduit for casting directors all over the world who call looking for actors for films and stage. Our staff and artists have moved all over the world as well, and continue to create and teach what inclusion is in their daily practice.

Full inclusion is also different from the older term 'mainstreaming.' Mainstreaming is an educational term from the mid-1970s that meant disabled young people were taken out of special homes, schools and programs for the disabled, and were 'mainstreamed' like 'normal' kids into regular activities, *but* (and here's the kicker) they were mainstreamed into those activities in separate small groups of disabled people within the bigger group, doing separate activities. Many artists disabled from birth have found themselves isolated, not only from performing, but from nearly every other aspect of life. Inclusive theatre doesn't do anything like mainstreaming, however it breaks down the walls of isolation. Everyone is in the same group, working on the same project. Period. That is inclusion. Inclusion implies a level of equal ownership within the project or endeavor. Inclusion is investment. Inclusion is ownership by the artist.

For the purposes of this book we will focus on our work with disabled artists as in theatre there are activities across the USA ensuring 'diversity and inclusion' but they historically and consistently focus on *every single other group* – except the disabled. The disabled are always a bridesmaid with all this activity, except for this book where they finally get to be the bride.

Also note that disability has as many variations as a rainbow. In fact, many more. Deaf is not the same as hard of hearing (and many deaf people do have residual hearing, another reason cochlear implants are so divisive within the Deaf community, as they remove any residual hearing when they are implanted). Low-level vision does not mean blind. Legally blind may not mean completely blind. Early CP or MS is very different from later stages CP and MS. The more you understand this the better you can progress in your work with artists with disabilities.

There are many reasons to be inclusive in the theatre such as simply having basic standards for any performer as a matter of equality. There is also the opportunity to create new performance or multimedia technology, create new performance styles, new acting styles, new staging concepts, new costume ideas, new scripts and writing styles, new lighting and sound and design ideology. Artists with disabilities are, by the nature of the beast, Olympic-class problem solvers and can teach you how to be one too. They have no choice but to find workarounds in their everyday life and bring those skills into rehearsals and performance. Creative problem solutions can also get you closer to tax incentives if you own a theatre space and want to refurbish it in order to become more accessible for your artists and/or audiences.

Our society tends to value people on their perceived ability to produce things, rather than their talent in producing meaningfulness in the lives of others. We are valued on how 'useful' we appear to be. If a disabled artist cannot immediately be perceived to be useful or to produce things in volume, money, activity or social popularity, they are traditionally discriminated against. However, you and your theatre or university can change all of that because the reality is that these ideas are a house of cards built on a foundation of air. The reality is that there are many reasons to work with disabled artists.

The first and best reason is that if you do not work with artists with disabilities you are missing out on a rich and varied talent pool, and that is both artistically amiss and box office stupid. You are not alone, Broadway took until 2015 to finally have an actor in a wheelchair grace its stage (and by that I mean a real actor who was really in a wheelchair playing a person in a wheelchair, not a box office name who is non-disabled playing a role in a wheelchair). Why did it take even Broadway so long, and why are they still falling behind? Why are they still not actively tracking and casting the disabled artists who should be working? Because of the habit of ignoring artists with disabilities and some very outdated societal misconceptions.

The most standard misconceptions people have about disability and inclusion and why they are wrong

You have to be extra nice to disabled people and cannot ever get mad or fire them.

Sounds silly and simplistic, right? However, until we stop treating artists with disabilities as if they are made of glass we are wasting our time and theirs. All the artists who work with me adhere to the same standards and if you do not, you get fired – yes, even if you are disabled. "But you can't fire me, I'm disabled, you need me!" a young man yelled at me once. "If you weren't disabled and did what you did, I would fire you. You do not get special treatment because you are disabled. I do not need anyone that bad." I replied. He wasn't fired because he was disabled, he was fired because he was a lazy and obnoxious actor who did not adhere to professional and union standards. This also goes for intellectual or developmental disabilities. Speak to artists with all disabilities clearly and preferably in a quiet space and continue until you know they get what you need them to understand. I have always found that developmental or intellectual disabilities have no bearing on intelligence or artistic talent so be certain to not treat them as such. Do not talk down. Talk with.

It is unbelievably hard to work with a disabled person because they need so many more 'things' than a non-disabled person.

What 'things' disabled artists are supposed to need above and beyond what non-disabled artists need is, you guessed it, nothing really. If there is anything extra like medicines, extra liquids, special transportation or anything else they will often usually arrange all of that themselves and never bother you with it. This saddens me in that they do not need to be so grateful to work that they do not want to bother me or the stage manager, but that often is the case.

I welcome the opportunity to know their needs as it helps me to know them both as people and artists. It also helps me to think of ways to incorporate their needs into the show, if we can, so it all becomes even easier and truer. Why not have it timed out so that they take their meds onstage as part of the play? Why not have them clean a prosthesis as an onstage action? It can all be made to work within the life of any play. In truth I usually have non-disabled actors who are much higher maintenance than the disabled actors.

If you do one play with one actor of color or one person in a wheelchair then you are inclusive and you are done.

Wrong. In the world of inclusion, one-offs do not count. You do not get to do a token casting and call yourself inclusive. If you have done that, shame on you. It disrespects the actor, you, the audience and the play and it is not inclusive and everyone knows it. Your audience may applaud, but they know you are cheating. Stop kidding yourself if you think casting one dark-skinned man in a show means you are 'diverse' as well – you are not. If you commit to being diverse and inclusive then do it, seriously. No more lip-service.

There is only one kind of wheelchair.

This sounds amusing in that non-wheelchair users never think about things like this. But let me tell you there are as many different wheelchairs as there are people who use them, and each one is an extension of the body of the individual who uses it. Do not assume that one person you know with a wheelchair has the same wheel width, weight or mobility as the other people you know in wheelchairs. There are manual chairs, electric chairs, racing chairs, extra-wide, lightweight, heavy-duty, antimicrobial, recliners – whew! Each one has different measurements, mobility realities, weights and lengths. We once had a co-producer of a show book our performances in a space he knew one of our actors who was a wheelchair user could fit. That was great except that our stage manager was also in a wheelchair that would not fit in that space. Our co-producer himself was disabled, although not in a wheelchair, so he just did not think it through thoroughly (which also emphasizes that just because a person is disabled does not mean they immediately understand all other disabilities by osmosis). Know who is involved with the show and know the technical specifications that come along with each person. If you do not know – ask. Anyone who uses a wheelchair generally knows what their measurements are, so just ask.

It is especially hard to work with deaf or blind artists.

Much of these types of misconceptions are fear based. If you do not speak out loud then I feel uncomfortable, if you are blind then I feel weird and do not know if I should look at you. I often get asked about how to cue deaf or blind actors to come onstage or to follow others who may be speaking dialogue. There are many ways to cue deaf actors like just tapping them on the arm or giving them a peephole to watch for a visual cue or having an onstage actor wave their arm, thus disrupting a beam of light that the deaf actor backstage sees. Vibratory cues are very useful as both deaf and blind actors are very adept at feeling vibrations. Have an onstage actor bang on something and then the deaf actor offstage can count to ten and enter. Have them count how many seconds after another actor enters until they enter and then use that. There are so many creative ways that are so simple it seems silly that this isn't being done more.

I am often asked, "But what if the actor who is deaf or blind is somewhere offstage where they cannot see any lights, or feel any vibrations or be cued by anyone at all? What do you do then?" And I reply, "Why would you put them in that place where they cannot get cued? What are you thinking? Who the heck is directing that play? Change it!" You *must* lead the way though. It really is very simple so do not complicate it. There is no rulebook, really, for ways to cue actors. If it works for you and for the artist then it will work for the audience.

A great many deaf actors are remarkable lip readers as well and can just watch the actors onstage and follow along. Even though many actors who are deaf read lips and even though I have a working knowledge of American Sign Language (ASL) I always have an interpreter when I direct deaf artists and would recommend all do the same unless they are fluent in ASL. It is my own failing that my

ASL is light years slower than my brain and I just simply cannot sign fast enough. I explain that to the deaf artists and apologize sincerely (because it is my fault) and then introduce my interpreter. I have been lucky to have two of the finest people I know act as my directing interpreters, Pamela O. Mitchell and Bram Weiser. Bram has become my go-to 'director' interpreter over time and when I do act onstage I try to only have Pamela co-play me or interpret for me. They get my rhythms and my quirks. They are the best.

My company did ASL work and had interpreted full performances and reading series from the beginning in 2001 with our projects for many years and had our own troupe of two wonderful interpreters at our core, Pamela (who now runs our ASL projects) and Gerald, 'terps' we called them. We would sit and work our way through the text with the playwright and actors and make sure that what they were signing was what we all wanted to say (as often the intended meaning is different than what is being verbalized).

One day someone asked me how come it was that all our terps were black? That caught me totally off guard, "Are they?" I replied, stymied. It had never crossed my mind what color they both were, just that they were part of our team and we could not create without them. I just never thought of them in terms of color, much as I do not think of folks in term of their disability, yet all the while I am very conscious of the disability as something of a technical issue. It is a fine line we walk, I suppose, but walking it with an honest purpose is what we need to do.

Alright, but what about folks who may be both deaf *and* blind? How do you work with or for them? Well, I have not had the chance yet to have an artist work with us who is both deaf *and* blind but we have had many audience members over the years who fit the bill. They do not just appear at performances, they always call way ahead of time. They always gave us a heads-up way before the performance they were attending and then we brought in very special interpreters for each of the audience members (as each deaf/blind audience member must have their own interpreter signing into their palm like Helen Keller was signed to) and after a pre-show tactile tour of the set (they get to feel any important props and get a bit of stage orientation and information) and any pre-show information they might need to know given to their interpreters, they and their personal interpreters were seated where it worked best for the interpreters and we went on with the show.

Did it cost a bit and take some organizing to bring in those interpreters? Yes. But they also cut their costs in half for us to help out and the overall cost was absorbed just fine. It was worth doing it because it is our mission statement that all should have access to live theatre.

Many theatres do not make any provisions for the deaf/blind audience member, so when they do find something they can attend, and a company that will welcome them, it is enormously fulfilling for them and for us. They are a 'part of' something, they are part of the creation and the performance and are not on the outside looking in. For the actors in the show, disabled and non-disabled, meeting with the deaf/blind audience members after the show and talking with them is a new way for them to see the impact their art has on an audience. It allows the artist to understand that their art has impacted someone who cannot hear them or see them. Think about that again.

The actor discovers that they have affected an audience member who cannot see or hear them.

This opens an actor's mind to all sorts of nuances and possibilities and the power of their work. Performance means power. For disabled artists many times there is a struggle with the dichotomy of being watched. They are oftentimes watched and/or stared at in life and have in many cases grown used to or calloused by the ever present gaze of the public because of their disability. Then we can explore new forms of 'seeing' disability and understanding the dynamics of 'the gaze' or 'the stare' when disability meets art and audience. Imagine the power and transformative change the work onstage brings when the eyes of others become a pleasing and empowering experience. Then to doubly realize that you can impart pain and pleasure to an audience without even being seen or heard at all? Wow. Why would you not want to be a part of that?

LGBTQIA artists who are disabled (or not) make it all about the sex and gender issues as well as being disabled and it gets very messy and embarrassing.

It is amusing how our assumptions keep us from being creative and block us from the LGBTQIA community as well. The transmutability of gender is another way societal norms are challenged, but for those with gender differences the reality is that they just want to be artists like everyone else. They have no more urge to discuss sex and gender and how it impacts their disability than anyone else. We just want to assume they do because then we can use that as an excuse and we do not have to deal with them. Frankly, they also just want to pee when and where they need to pee. The only bathroom issue that matters is if they need an accessible one and will their wheelchair fit? So, let's stop assuming, stop the debate about what is or is not in people's pants, and invite them in as artists and designers and students and actors and get back to the business of creating art. It is only messy if *you* make it messy.

It costs more money to be inclusive because of all of the added expenses.

Again, this is never fully thought out by the nay-sayer. What expenses? Extra rehearsal time? No. Massive transportation costs for Access-A-Ride or some other service? No. Extra set pieces or costuming? No. Extra snacks? There is no real extra. We work in only accessible spaces and sometimes that might be a bit more expensive, but that is our plan to do that from the beginning of any production (and already budgeted) so once the artists are cast there is no added expense at all, except perhaps occasionally building a wheelchair ramp or having a deaf/blind interpreter (which is very rare). This 'high costs' issue is a pure fallacy and again a prime example of ways we block ourselves from involving these groups out of fear or ignorance.

Because an artist is disabled it means they have less talent or are less able to communicate their talent and so we must pity them as an audience.

This, this is a big one. Much of the time this misconception is given great weight. Unjustly so. I have in fact, found the opposite to be true most of the time. I have found that the pain and trials and mistreatment and having to fight to be heard and to be an artist has only served to make most artists with disabilities even more amazing and resilient. They bring with them a weight of having lived through something big and made it through it, and that is a lot more of a creative pot to dip into than an actor who just has lost their bus pass. Some disabled artists may have less training than non-disabled artists, but this is through no fault of their own. The fault lies in our educational system and the academics and recruiters who have closed minds.

The disabled artist is a person and has the same range of likes and dislikes and talents as those who are not disabled. Communication is easy once you start. However, be logical. Not all blind people read braille; not all people who use wheelchairs play wheelchair basketball; and not all deaf people read lips. Not all artists with disabilities have a Juilliard background. But this does not mean they do not have talent and cannot communicate. Talk with them about things you talk about with other folks – weather, sports, politics, food, sex, politics, what you did today. Given the safe space to grow and a disciplined and professional example to follow, these artists will wow you, the other cast members, themselves and the audience.

Working with service animals is disruptive and dangerous and messy.

We have had the extreme joy of working with three service dogs and one other dog (as an actor) in our seventeen seasons and let me tell you they are great. I wish all the actors behaved as well as the service animals! Yes, wee-wee pads are good to have around, but their owner will bring them. If you are working with a service dog in a show you need to discuss this in a cast meeting and set the rules.

Standard rules are when the dog is in a harness it is working and you leave it alone no matter how cute it is. Once the actor or designer and dog are on break the actor will remove the dog from harness if it is their choice. Some artists with service dogs want the dog 'on' at all times and so the dog is always working. Other artists may give the dog breaks out of harness so that the cast and crew can pet and meet them. It is always good to have a doggie bowl and a mat or blanket available if needed for water for the dogs as well, but again usually the artist will provide everything for their animal.

The one overwhelming rule about dogs onstage, service dogs or dogs who are cast in a role (like our lovely Clare who was in *The Cherry Orchard*), is that once that dog goes onstage you can forget about the audience paying attention to anything else for about three to five minutes. Dogs will always steal the show no matter what theatre or show they are in.

The reasons theatres, college training programs or practitioners are not inclusive

1   They are afraid – you are not like me so I am afraid of you.

2   There is some ignorance of the reality of the work – I assume it is expensive, time-consuming and hard to work with you and I will not do any research to change my assumptions.

3   There need to be guidebooks, guidelines, checklists and practical help like this book to assist in dispelling antiquated notions and ideas about inclusion.

4   They have misconceptions about the process of inclusion and assume it must happen overnight and on a large scale. Not true. So, start slowly, engage a blind actor for a season. Inclusion doesn't mean you have to have every LGBTQIA, person of color and disabled artist in your state working with you by next week. Take your time, it is a process, but do it.

5   They feel safe producing what they do, and do not move beyond their safe zone. Maybe you produce musicals with extensive dancing and singing and cannot for the life of you see how you could work a disabled artist into that. Then start with a designer, or a stage manager who is disabled and do that for a season. Once you see how easy it is you will get it. The physicality of dance is an amazing realm that you can explore together. One of my dreams is to choreograph a tap sequence with up to five amputee dancers, utilizing tap, clapping of hands and snapping of fingers – now that is great theatre!

6   They do not understand accessibility issues and fear it will cost money to make everything accessible. Some places are more accessible than you think. Elevators are the main tough spots. Then hallways, can they be negotiated in a wheelchair? Ramps are easy to build, even to Americans with Disabilities Act (ADA) specifications (I have lost track of how many ramps we have built or carried or stored over the years) and once they are in place you are good to go. Chances are that if you walk through your space you will realize, "OK, wheelchairs will never get through, but that actor with the prosthetic leg we could hire him, he was so talented and we do not have many stairs." Work with who you are able to, but stop stopping yourself from working.

7   They fear loss of their funders, audiences, board members, etc. if they become inclusive. The fear of monetary loss is a very real fear, but if you lose a donor (and really how petty would that be to withdraw funds because an artist who is disabled is hired?) I can guarantee that you will gain five more who will be delighted to fund accessible needs and disabled artists. Perhaps you have an older, powerful board member who wants what they want onstage and they control the purse strings. Hmmm, perhaps that board member needs to be told that a younger, richer board member can be found (and they can be) who is more on board with the twenty-first century reality. Appeal to a stodgy board member that they have a chance to be on the front line of new artistic expression and let them mull that one over. You might be surprised at what they say. They are on your board hopefully because they are smart, so challenge them.

8   What about audiences? In seventeen seasons we have never lacked for audiences and never had audiences leave due to a disabled artist, actor, stage manager, crew person or designer. Ever. Remember twenty percent of the US is disabled today, think about that. *Twenty percent.* That is a huge audience base just waiting for theatres to say, "We welcome you, we want to work with and for you." This doesn't count their family and friends either!

All these misconceptions can be dealt with. But what about the wrong reasons to be inclusive? Isn't being inclusive great, no matter what? No. Not if done for the wrong reasons.

The wrong reasons to be inclusive

1   Money or some immediate grant opportunity or outside influence. Let's say a sizeable grant comes up, but you must have a disabled person in a cast so you use one disabled person in one thing to get the grant and then drop the artist after that. Not only is it morally questionable, but the backlash from the disabled community (and I would hope the arts community in general) will be endless. Also you will never get that grant again. Do not even think about doing it.

2 Press or social media gratification. Again, it is not worth it and if the press realizes you are doing it for the press, they can turn on you too and that is never good. Do not work with artists who are disabled for press or media attention.
3 For one role in one play where they must have a person who is disabled and there is absolutely no way around that so they do it 'just this once.' You cannot un-open that door. Once you open up to working with artists with disabilities then do it. Do not do a one-off. It disrespects you, the playwright, your audience, the artists and your community.

Again, commit to doing it and doing it for the right reasons. Start small by adding a disability consultant to your board, add a disabled playwright or a dramaturg who is blind. Hire a stage manager in a wheelchair and see where you go from there. Have someone like me walk through your theatre and make access suggestions or discuss your season with you. The choices we make define us, and you *can* redefine yourself, your theatre, your university. Even Deaf West in Los Angeles and the New York City based Theater Breaking Through Barriers were not trying to be fully inclusive until maybe 2012. Before that they worked with deaf and blind artists respectively and exclusively. However, they got it, they understood that paradigm shifts were coming and they both changed their mandates, mission statement and casting. Your group, university or theatre can do the same.

Case Study 2: Stage Manager in a Wheelchair, Nicu's Spoon Theater, Long Island City, New York

History

Over our seasons my company, Nicu's Spoon, has worked with tons of wheelchairs and tons of wheelchair users. We are familiar with probably every type of chair. The toughest ones are the electric wheelchairs for two reasons. They are heavy. (We had an artist once who called his electric wheelchair King Kong.) I mean 200–300 pounds without the person in them (and most of the time the person in an electric chair is more physically fragile than someone rushing around in a manual chair doing wheelies) and they are run by a battery, which must be recharged. A vital tip to remember is to have a backup battery charged at all times if you use an electric wheelchair onstage or offstage for an actor or staff member, just in case. So, we were pretty well versed with chairs – for our actors.

In 2015 we hired a young assistant stage manager (ASM), Marco Naranjo, who was in an electric wheelchair. Although we had once had an ASM in a manual chair for a reading series, an ASM in an electric wheelchair was a new one for us. It was a highly complicated show with twenty-six actors aged five to seventy-five, eight musical numbers and probably one-third or more of the cast had disabilities of varying kinds. There were nearly sixty costume changes, sixty light changes, ninety plus props and about forty multimedia slides throughout the show. We had the best stage manager ever (Juni Li was later to win a NYITA in New York City for her amazing work on this production of *Red Noses*) and another ASM, Felicia Castaldo, who was the backstage and onstage ASM.

Marco was a new graduate out of Pace University and was like a sweet puppy, eager to learn, lamenting that he couldn't carry a lot on his lap while driving his wheelchair around, but that was alright. The problems came as we readied to open the show in the wonderful Secret Theater in Long Island City, five minutes from Manhattan. In the past this theatre had been one of the rare theatres to have their light booth on the ground floor, but in renovating they had moved everything way above the stage and up a tight, rickety ladder. The other ASM, Felicia, was the backstage and onstage ASM (having been worked into the show), but Marco had been intended to be in the booth running sound, while Juni ran lights and multimedia. We loaded into the theatre, found out where the new light booth was and went, "Oh boy."

Plan

How could we get Marco up there? Did his chair have to go up there too? How did we solve it? Not just solve it but solve it so that the tech ran smoothly, Marco did not get hurt or mangled and we didn't spend tons of money building anything. If you think you have it figured out then re-figure it out but put Marco in a lightweight manual chair, not a 300-pound chair, and deal with the same problem. There are two solutions for this. Test yourself.

See Chapter 16 for further details of this case study.

3

VOCABULARY AND PERCEPTION

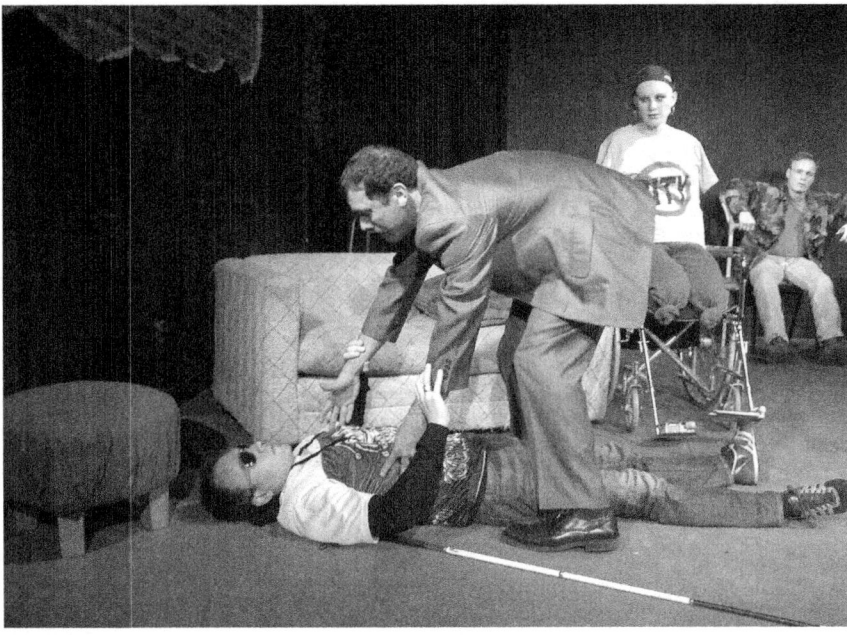

Figure 3.1   *Kite Cut Loose in the Middle of the Sky* by David Greenberg, 2008. L to R Tim Romero, Leo Otero, Margaret Baker and Mark Armstrong. (Photograph courtesy of Nicu's Spoon Theater Company.)

Let's start by discussing people-first language (PFL, also sometimes called person-first language). The basic idea of PFL (which began to be used around 1989 starting with appearing in the National Affordable Housing Act) was to use a sentence structure that names the person first and the condition second, for example 'people with disabilities' rather than 'the disabled,' in order to emphasize that 'they are people first.' However, because English syntax normally places adjectives before nouns, we have to then insert relative clauses, replacing, e.g., 'asthmatic person' with 'a person who has asthma.' But the terms and the idea were mostly created and used initially by teachers, doctors, nurses, social workers and government professionals in order to be a type of etiquette for the non-disabled community and in the long run this usually does not work for the disabled community. PFL continues to be touted as the law of the land mostly due to educational literature and social services, but as the disabled community grows their disabilities are a source of identity and pride (and rightfully so) and identity-first language (IFL) is preferred by the majority. Those with disabilities have concerns about ableism and stereotyping and in the fields of special education and social work this has turned into a hegemonic policy of PFL, with special educators, social workers, academics and other non-disabled advocates often insisting on using PFL even when the people they work with prefer IFL.

Both usages will be found in this book, but the debate rages on. The most common disability model within the disabled community is the social/cultural model, which emanates from the idea that disability is a socio-political construct and that fears language and stereotypes are the real barriers to individuals with disabilities. Thus, IFL is gaining ground in popularity. We all take refuge in language and terms we are used to, and find comfort in them, but there are unmistakable signs the vocabulary around us is changing rapidly to match the disability rights movement.

For many, not all, PFL makes no sense. PFL would mean I would then say I am a person with womanhood. In Deaf culture (using capital D 'Deaf' to denote the culture/community and its members and the lower-case D 'deaf' to denote the audiological condition as is preferred in the Deaf community) PFL has long been rejected. Instead, Deaf culture uses Deaf-first language since being culturally deaf is a source of positive identity and pride. ASL, the language of the Deaf, means *American* Sign Language and that does mean that there are other 'SL' languages like British Sign Language (BSL) and Cyprus/Cypriot Sign Language (CSL). There are well over 125 sign languages in the world.

Well-known autism activist Jim Sinclair also rejects PFL, as do many in the autistic community, because saying 'person with autism' suggests that autism can be separated from the person. Most blind and mobility-impaired disability advocates also reject PFL, defining themselves as 'disabled people' and the 'disability' is the discrimination they face as a result of their impairments. I ask what artists themselves prefer and the vast majority dislike PFL. If you use PFL, check and see if those you work with prefer it. If they do not then do not use it. Simple. I know what my preference is, I prefer to call them an actor or director or by their first name (and often am taken to task for forgetting to say what their disability is), but I ultimately do what the artists prefer.

I would not tell another person what language to use as this continues to be an extremely debated issue even within the disability community and especially the disability theatre community, and even by state or region. Take care to apologize if someone prefers PFL, even if you do not. Using both PFL and IFL is the way to work, depending upon whom you speak with. This same care should be taken with members of the LGBTQIA community as some may be non-binary, gay, transgendered, gender-fluid and may identify with the use of specific pronouns.

The disability rights movement is about accommodating the differences, not erasing, hiding or apologizing for them. The impairment is not the actual physical or medical 'disability.' The impairment may be a degenerative back disease, the disability is being unable to get up the stairs of the library in your wheelchair. The true disability is the actual inability to function in a world that is not set up for you. Thus, the social model of disability understands the problem of disabled people as being in the social environment, not in their impairment. By promoting the social model of disability (and placing emphasis on changing society rather than the individual) disability advocates and activists have been able to demand equal opportunities and rights. If we think of disability as something that is imposed upon people with impairments due to the structure of their environment then we direct attention towards removing barriers in society (attitudinal, economic and political as well as the physical) to facilitate access for disabled people. Thus, the linguistic practices of society must be set up for those with disabilities as well.

On the average, most artists and people with disabilities do not think of themselves as activists and may want nothing to do with being one. Overall, the artists simply want to be hired and trained and paid and called by name.

Again and again I hear the same incorrect ideas about what it is like to work with disabled artists and many of the questions are very basic. "Well, how do you talk to them?" (As if they are human beings is always a good bet.) "How do you ask about their disability? Should you ask about it?" (Of course, you should if it is pertinent to the play, their work, their stamina, their performance or course work in school, etc.) In general, it is not your right to ask about it if you do not need to. It is not a mystery you need to solve and it is not their job to explain it to you. They are artists and people, not individual educators for you. Ask about it if you need to, with care and humor. It is not as if the asking about it makes them aware of it. ("What?! I have a handicap? Are you kidding me?! How could I have missed that?!") If you do not ask them and you really should be asking them then you are either overly nervous or very lazy. "What should you call them?" I usually call them by name. Ask them. Make the effort. But only if it really matters. Many times it simply doesn't matter at all, you just think it does.

If an artist prefers PFL, I am supportive of that as it is not my place how any or every disabled artist feels about words. However, the vocabulary we use, the terminology, is important to all of us, because words reflect the continuing societal attitudes and beliefs. Disabled people have historically and traditionally been 'labeled' by medical, welfare, social and charitable organizations and described in terms of what is 'wrong' with them.

Talleri McRae, a wonderful disability advocate, writer and consultant and new mom, has a presentation of the history of disability and language, highlights being 'handicapped' literally taken from the term 'cap in hand' with the idea that the disabled held their cap out and begged for assistance. Or the god-awful cheery 'Handi-capable!' which is the non-disabled person's way of assuring disabled folks that, "You are just as good as us, Hon!" Ugh.

As Talleri will tell you, "The difference between a disabled and a non-disabled experience is not fortune, it's privilege." Imagine being denied the privilege of being able to enter your own school, your classroom, an audition room, your apartment complex, a restroom.

A recent movement in the USA, following on the heels of a vibrant, growing and political disability culture and the brilliant and up-front movie festivals 'Diss-This' and 'ReelAbilities' in New York City and expounded on by disability advocates/activists Lawrence Carter-Long and Christine DeZinno Bruno is about just naming it what it is. Saying it. #saytheword, #Disability. You can say it too, I know you can. The current reclaiming of the word 'cripple' and 'crip,' similar to the gay community reclaiming the word 'queer' for their own re-defining and ownership, connects these terms to a new activism and identity that is edgier and does not take "No" for an answer any longer. Thus a term like 'crip face' or 'cripping up' becomes equatable with 'blackface' or the more common term in usage in 2016, the 'whitewashing' of roles in Hollywood.

Terms like 'differently abled' (which I admit to using for about six months) or worse yet 'handi-capable' are perceived as patronizing by the disabled community. For example, referring to a person as 'confined to a wheelchair' or a 'victim' of a particular condition is emotionally loaded, patronizing and biased (and also darn wrong as many folks in wheelchairs can get out of them fast and kick your butt before you can blink an eye). This language perpetuates outdated ideas about people with disabilities as subjects to be pitied and not taken seriously, rather than being seen in the same light as people without disabilities. Thus, this language separates them from the society and from you.

So, for me and me alone I simply call it like I see it. Disabled, uses a wheelchair, has a prosthetic leg, is an amputee, has CP, is autistic, is blind, is deaf, is a little person. Just say it. What do I really call disabled artists? I call them by name and rarely mention their disability at all. The top ten greatest hits on the 'do not use these terms so we can *all* be treated with respect' list are based on 'The Language of Disability: Dos and Don'ts' by inclusioninthearts.org

	Don't Use	*Do Use*
1	Wheelchair-bound/ confined to	Wheelchair user/uses a wheelchair/electric wheelchair, not electric chair.
2	Suffers from/afflicted with/crippled by	These terms make assumptions about how the disabled person feels about his/ her disability. Use 'has' and the name of condition (e.g., has cerebral palsy, has paraplegia, etc.).
3	The disabled/the blind/ the deaf	Always use as an adjective rather than a noun – disabled person, blind filmmaker, deaf man or woman.
4	Retarded/mentally retarded/retard	Intellectual disability; cognitive disability; developmental disability. When using these terms, however, it is important to understand the distinctions among them.
5	Handicapped (handicap)	In general: if you're not writing about sports, do not use it! Use disability, disabled person, person with a disability.
5a	Handicapped parking, restroom, etc.	Accessible parking, restroom, etc.
6	Midget/dwarf	Little person or short of stature; dwarf is acceptable only if the subject actually has dwarfism. Keep in mind: Anyone with dwarfism is a little person, but not every little person is a dwarf.
7	Deaf-mute/deaf and dumb	Deaf
	Hearing-impaired	Hard of hearing
8	Physically challenged/ differently abled	Avoid outdated or saccharine terms and euphemisms. Use disabled as an adjective (e.g., disabled sportscaster).
9	Overcoming/inspiring/ brave/courageous	Avoid patronizing and condescending descriptives – describe the person's accomplishments without value judgment or interpretation.
10	Special	Do not use when referring to disabled people.

Source: http://inclusioninthearts.org/faqs/the-language-of-disability-dos-and-donts/

Many phrases we might not think of as appropriate are perfectly acceptable, however. People who use wheelchairs do 'go for a walk.' It is perfectly acceptable to say to a person with a visual disability, "See you later," or to a deaf person, "Did you hear about…" People with disabilities really do not find common everyday phrases of this kind offensive and use them in conversation with each other all the time. It is only the non-disabled or TABs (temporarily able bodied) who worry about this being offensive. I know a wonderful little person artist who will tell you she is vertically challenged. I love that as it is very funny (and she is equally funny) and I love how she loves to take people aback with her humor. It wakes and shakes them up.

Many artists with disabilities and designers who have worked with my company for years will often spur questions from non-disabled newcomers. New members will ask me, "Well, how did they get disabled?" and sometimes I really do not know. I know they are and I know their current medical or physical and emotional issues and we work with that, but I do not always know the whole story of their particulars because I do not need to and it is not my inherent right to know. Unless of course I need to, or they need me to. If you need to know, ask. Just ask. If they need to tell you they will, but only if they know you will really hear them. So, you must, as director, producer, academic or advisor make yourself open to hearing them. I say a lot, "Whatever you want or need to tell me, I will listen and hear you." I mean that, and you must too.

Part of our labeling of the disabled artist also comes out historically in casting. Disabled actors are always cast as either the horribly and irredeemably evil one or more likely the saints, the loners, those touched by God, those with special powers, those who are good and honest and pure and then die so we can reflect on how they have enriched our lives. We can watch this then and feel inspired by their disability and uplifted by their sacrifice, much as we feel uplifted when the homecoming queen asks the autistic boy to the prom on YouTube.

The flip side of this saint/sinner labeling is what the disabled community themselves call the above asking the autistic boy to the prom 'inspiration porn.' The term inspiration porn was coined in 2012 by disability rights activist Stella Young. The term describes when people with disabilities are called inspirational solely or in part on the basis of their disability. This includes commercials and images that portray disabled people doing things that would be ordinary to the non-disabled but calling them 'inspirational' because the person doing them is disabled. For example, inspiration porn sometimes shames the viewer by showing a disabled person overcoming basic obstacles like tying their shoes, the implication then being that anyone less disabled has no excuse. Another very popular variant, which is all over social media, focuses on individuals doing something for people with disabilities, inviting them to the prom, suggesting that others should help too, centering attention on the helper as the hero, not on the disabled recipient.

In all cases, the non-disabled person is a hero and the disabled person gets treated similarly to a prop or as sweet, dumb folks to be pitied. That is not how they see themselves and we must stop placing them in these roles. Would we be as intrigued if the football player with Down's syndrome took pity on the pretty cheerleader and asked her out and filmed it for YouTube? Would we then call her 'so brave and inspiring' with a saccharine tone in our voice?

I personally adore casting disabled actors as villains, drug addicts, sex-fiends, rapists and killers. I also love to cast them in heroic leading roles. First, they rarely get to play the lead or villains so they love it and second the audience then has to come to a complete stop and re-think their own pre-packaged ideas about the 'instant sainthood' society labels the disabled with and that they have read about or seen on television or in films. I also love to cast disabled actors in roles where they have a disability that is not their natural one. Having three or four disabled artists in one show with each one playing a disability they do not have is a wonderful opportunity for each of them to grow as an artist and re-examine their own personal notions of being disabled.

Another way we must continue to cast disabled artists, and this is vital, are as sexual beings, lovers, parents (another ongoing societal misconception, as many disabled people are parents), those who get the prince or princess in the end, those who are sexy, those who love and are loved. Those who have sexual relations. This is another way society and casting de-humanize and de-sexualize disabled people as an entire community. But they do love, are loved in return and are sexy. They have sex and romance, they have children and are sensual beings. Cast them accordingly.

I have known and continue to know many artists with disabilities from all over the world and let me be the first one to burst the misconception bubble, they are not all saints. Truth. In fact, there are a few I do not like at all. Just like, oh, non-disabled people. Some people are great and some are not and if you are lucky like I have been then you will get to work with and know the best of the best. So let's move on from the 'saints or sinners' model of typecasting.

Case Study 3: Disabled Artist as Villain, Nicu's Spoon Theater, New York City

History

In 2007 my company had managed to move into an actual space in New York City, a true miracle considering the expense of buying or renting anything in that city. We renovated and made a small theatre on 38th Street. (Although we did not know the future five years would involve many elevator outages and carrying wheelchairs and artists up the stairs while singing lustily!)

For our first production in the space we chose *Richard III* and as I had just the prior year met and made fast friends with actor/writer/playwright and activist Henry Holden (who passed away in early 2016 and the world suffered a huge loss) I offered him the lead role of Richard. Henry had contracted polio as a child and was in his forties at the time, he walked with arm crutches and his lower half was smaller than his upper. Funny, charismatic and smart like crazy, he was great fun and we went to work. I produced and hired a promising and talented young female director, Heidi Lauren Duke, to direct it. About halfway through the rehearsal process I was let in on a problem that was happening. Henry couldn't memorize some of his lines. Hmmm, *some* of his lines?

I set forth to figure this out as he had starred in many other things in the past and didn't seem to have issues with lines. After watching rehearsals and talking with him I realized he was having what I termed a 'physical disconnect.' If he stood still (as Richard does when he 'monologues' to the audience and lets them in on his plans) he remembered all his lines. However, if he started moving around the stage in complicated scenes his body demanded his attention and his brain lost his lines. This is a three-act play with a lot of dialogue and about half (the monologues to the audience) he had memorized, but no matter what we worked on, the minute he moved he lost the lines. And we were about one week from production when we really knew we had to do something. Tickets were selling like hotcakes and Henry's movement was all perfect physically, he just couldn't talk and move together. The director, brave girl, was beside herself and looked at me like, "It is your company. Fix it!" and rightfully so.

Plan

So, what did I do? How to make the show go on, with Henry, with no ticket losses, with something inventive that we could do quickly that did not require recasting or time to re-block the entire show? Something that was, in reviews, hailed as a radical and brilliant production choice? The answer may surprise you.

See Chapter 16 for further details of this case study.

4

RECRUITING AND FINDING ARTISTS

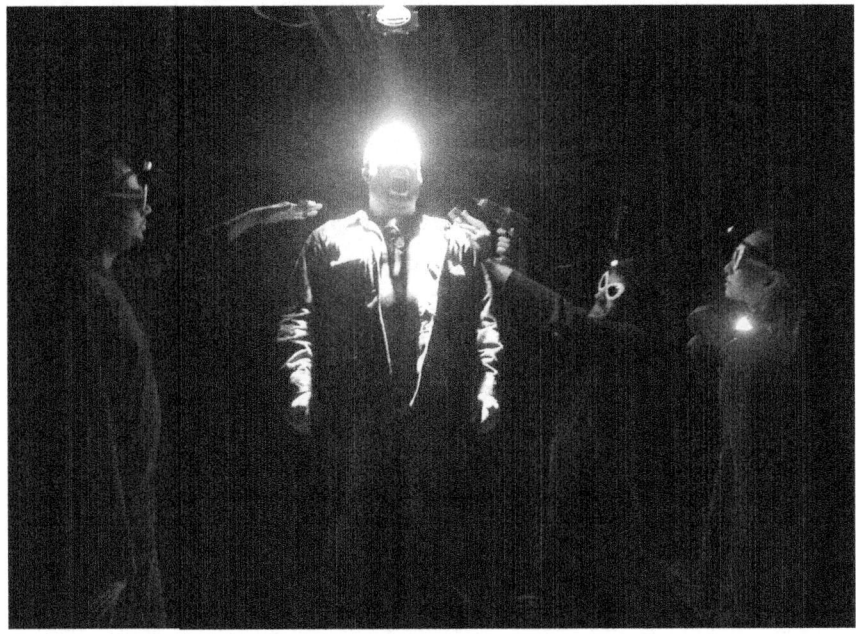

Figure 4.1   *Tales of the Lost Formicans* by Constance Congdon, 2007. L to R Dirk Smile,
Michael Hartney, Russell Waldman and Jovinna Chan. (Photograph
courtesy of Nicu's Spoon Theater Company.)

Recruiting and actively finding artists with disabilities and technical
staff can be very hard, and even more difficult if you are not in a
large and international city like New York. The first five or six years
of my company producing I looked high and low and often talked
with artists who had stopped working because of their disability
(either a disability coming later in life or a degenerative one). I
would find myself talking them back into working, but not without

some suspicion. We had to prove ourselves, that we were not just doing a one-off and that we really had a long-term and thorough commitment to this varied community. I confronted then, and still confront at rare times, the idea that perhaps I have ulterior motives myself in working with these disabled artists. Perhaps I want to use them to get grants. Even if there were enough grants to make that our motivation, it still wouldn't be as important as the experience, community and creation of art together. Any suspicion you are met with is normal and you simply must be persistent and transparent about your thoughts and intentions. You must learn about and discover this community. Make an investment in order to begin. Importantly, *specifically* include disability in the list of 'diversities' welcome to apply (beyond women, minorities, etc.). Say and use the word.

Making an investment also applies not only to universities who wish to recruit but also to conferences, symposiums, consortiums and so forth. Every year many disabled activists, artists and writers apply for or are asked to apply for large conferences as presenters, lecturers and the like. However ninety-five percent of these symposiums and conferences not only make no provision for accessibility needs (for the very people they want to lecture at their conferences), they are also quick to let all potential presenters know they must foot the bill for all expenses. In what ways does this bad planning encourage more participation? Before you can think perhaps the conferences themselves do not have funds I can point out that the Kennedy Center, in fact, sponsors one of these conferences and still requires that the lecturers pay for themselves.

Making inroads into these communities, whether to find audiences or artists, is much more than simply stating you want to do a show for or with them or you want them to come and lecture for you. You must possess the right knowledge and language, terminology, comprehension of various disabilities, an understanding of hot button issues in the community, an active knowledge of disability onstage and disabled artists onstage, a commitment to accessible work, active board or company members who are members of these communities and an investment in audience development (as opposed to offering them a show as a one-off). This is a solid commitment and for you, I hope, a long-term one.

You and your company must be willing to make a monetary, structural, programmatic, decision-making (read board and staff members) and artistic investment into the disability groups and community. There may also be suspicion if you do not 'present' as a disabled person in your outward appearance, and this too is normal. Simply keep talking and investing your time, planning, energy and artistic choices and the truth of your intentions will out.

You will always want to work with experienced artists, however you will also work with new artists with little or no experience, and we are fully aware of the lack of formal training programs focused on the disabled artists. We also love, as must you, to bring artists back to the arts who have left because of a disability but have some solid training and credits. We always aim for working with professionals or training or interning new folks to be professionals.

Many of these artists have been in an atmosphere in their life and in school or even around their own family where their voices are ignored, squashed or denied. Perhaps they have spent years trying to be heard by people who simply assume they have no voice at all. They really do rely on us as teachers, colleagues and directors to provide a stage where they can find their voice and we both can overthrow the cultural norms that make our society run on unfairly.

My company was always on the hunt when we first started in 2001, whether it was for new board members or for artists to work with. After about year five we were able to relax a bit and let artists come to us. In 2008 Screen Actors Guild (SAG), Actors Equity Association (AEA) and American Federation of Television and Radio Artists (AFTRA) launched the 'I Am PWD' campaign to promote inclusion and accessibility in arts and film work for people with disabilities. I was lucky enough to be able to speak at all the union offices at that time about our company and invite new artists in. That and good public relations and reviews and some extra good word of mouth and a lot of community networking also helped us to make contacts and inroads to finding more wonderful artists.

We learned that when looking for artists with disabilities it is not enough just to put out an open audition call. Sometimes you must contact many of your local groups like churches, community and neighborhood centers, social media groups, acting schools and websites, disability groups, schools, training centers, veterans' organizations, hospital outpatient groups, other theatres. Contact them and offer to put up a flyer with information for what you need, when your show rehearses, when auditions are, when it is performing and what roles are available. Nowadays social media and online platforms are the norm for your audition calls as well.

Also in your audition ad mention salary, contract, union house or even a stipend if that is all you can provide. We *always* pay something to every actor, whether they are union or not. It may (in some leaner years) be only transportation reimbursement, but we always pay our artists. Getting money for designing or acting or writing a play is an enormously empowering thing. It says, "You and your work have value and I recognize that." For countless artists over the years we have been the first people who have paid them for their art and it does matter. You can see it on their face. (A tip: Even if you are a very small company, always pay by check of course as you need your paper trail, but many artists who have gotten their first check from us over the years frequently copy and frame it!)

You must also, when recruiting artists, ask clearly for what you want. So, then you must also know what you want. If you know you are stuck in a performance space for your season that has no elevator access for wheelchairs, then say so and decide what kinds of disabilities you could work with and ask specifically for that in your recruiting efforts.

If you want to start out only working with deaf or blind artists then be upfront about that in your search for them. If you work with deaf artists, please have a Director of ASL (DASL – pronounced dazzle) and commit to it. Commit to having a person who is the final say in the ASL decisions to be made in the text. Do not fall into the trap of signed English (SE) or signed exact English (SEE) which is a sentence signed in grammatically correct English and has *nothing* to do with the beauty and imagery and syntax and grammar of ASL. ASL is a real language and to use SEE as a vehicle for communication with a deaf person is the mental equivalent of using pig Latin while speaking.

You may have to actively search for the artists you need because some of them may have been very broken down, by their job, family, society, their ongoing pain and medical needs, their own fears, but it is worth it when you find them. Frequently I would find myself on someone's couch in the early years, talking someone back into theatre after they had withdrawn from it. A new or even degenerative disability doesn't remove the fact that they are still an artist and it is the artist you are looking for.

With the search for deaf artists I have been very fortunate to have had the help of the Deaf community and many interpreters in New York City and they have always put me in touch with wonderful artists. One of the times an artist really impressed not only me, but the cast and the audience was in the case of Shira Grabelsky. I had been emailing her in 2007 as we did our first season in our first permanent space on 38th Street. We had already created a new kind of performance style called co-playing and she had heard of us in the Deaf community.

My thoughts behind creating co-playing was to enable not only deaf and hearing actors to act together, but to be able to present the project to a deaf and hearing audience simultaneously. Thus, one deaf and one hearing actor would simultaneously act the same role at the same time. In co-playing, for example, the acting pairs might move together or may be on opposite sides of the stage but they are always connected visually and in similar dress. Once the audience gets the concept of, "Oh those two are the same person!" (after about the first five minutes) then we are off and running. Notions that the speaking actors are primary or the 'lead' are discarded rapidly and frequently the signing artist takes the lead. The actors may also trade off, with the speaking actor signing with the deaf actor at a particular specific moment. The process is very text and image based and defies the expectations of both the text and the conventional roles deaf and hearing actors have traditionally taken.

We were doing our second co-played piece in 2007, a British play called *Kosher Harry* and eventually Shira Grabelsky was co-cast, along with one of my favorite actresses in New York City, Wynne Anders, as 'The Old Lady.' They were as unalike as could be, these two, one sixty years old, the other twenty-five, one a little person and one a bigger person, one deaf and one hearing (yes, Shira was a deaf little person, those two disabilities often go hand in hand more than people realize) but they were a wild and rowdy twosome onstage and they developed an almost psychic connection in that it seemed Shira never needed to be cued into when Wynne was speaking, she just seemed to sense it. Wynne seemed to know how to pace and breathe so that she never pushed or rushed Shira signing. Their sense of ribald humor matched well and the absolute show-stopping great moment of the entire play was when they both did a 'hootchy-kootchy, hot-mama dance' to tremendous and screaming applause from the audience. Before you even ask, yes, they did indeed dance to music and in sync and they were marvelous!

I am always open to finding artists wherever and whenever I can and you must be as well. My company hosted a New York discussion panel on disabled artists in 2007 and a tall skinny young man with a few missing fingers and maybe a glass eye showed up. He sat attentively in the audience and as I sneakily looked at him I realized he had (and pardon to Stephen King) a 'shine.' He glowed with good will, laughed readily and had an innate sweetness. I made it my mission to meet him and learn about him. Sammy Mena, one of my favorite actors in the world, became a company member that night (although he didn't know it till maybe a few months later) and he has played villains, animals, women, brilliant doctors and zombies for us over the years. Our audiences adore him, he went to an Off-Broadway contract with us and got rave reviews in the New York City papers and he is absolute magic and I adore working with him. (Plus he does have an assortment of cool glass eyes he can use! One has a happy face! Awesome!)

My point is that I could have simply been in 'panel host' mode the night I met Sammy, but I wasn't, I was (and really still am) always actively looking for artists. (I also confess that every building I enter, probably for the rest of my life, I immediately assess for accessibility in every single way.) Artists can be found many places besides audition settings so be certain to search widely and go into your daily life paying attention.

I actively, consciously and constantly search out ignored and marginalized artists, many of whom have removed themselves from the arts as a result of being disabled. So should you. So should your organization or university. We have disabled board members (the wonderful author, Daniel Tammett, who has autism, is on our board) and always have disabled staff and designers and playwrights so for us this is a true commitment. We are also actively committed to all colors, races, genders, ages and the entire rainbow of the LGBTQIA community.

In late 2013 I was in pre-production for a play that I knew would be followed and filmed from start to finish by a documentary crew and director. In truth they were with my company for nearly eight months and became a de facto 'family' to us all in the company. I put out an audition call and had been talking to a funny and very smart actor by the name of Anthony M. Lopez. Part of his interview and audition was filmed and appears in the documentary made about my company, Nicu's Spoon, called *Two and Twenty Troubles* and he told me that he really had backed away from acting for quite a few years although he had good training and experience, that he kind of felt like he didn't know where to start or how to present himself in a world increasingly ruled by reality TV stars and not talent. I cast him in *The Cherry Orchard* as Lopakhin and he was amazing, really just a lovely and fearless actor. Since our show ended he has begun working on his own productions, has done tons of print work, television, Subway, S'well and Heineken commercials (and his Broad City cameo as 'leg guy' is hysterical) and he is actively out in the world, creating and doing. I do not take a bit of credit, it is all him. But I am so delighted that we have been part of the jumpstart to his journey back into acting. The world needs his talent and humor desperately.

I cast actors who are the best for the role, to make a point, show them off in a new way, challenge them and shake up preconceived notions of a play, a role, a stereotype or a stodgy idea that the audience has. How else can we reflect current society? How else can we grow and change and think? And is that not what theatre should be doing? And for the love of theatre and all that is holy, if you do have a play with a disabled role of any kind in it – *cast a disabled actor* (even if he has a different disability than the role!). When the actor comes to curtain call and remains blind or in a wheelchair then your work has a social, personal and emotional impact on the audience. The actor does not hop out of their chair and do a jig at curtain call, thus erasing the power of everything that has just transpired onstage. At least for now until things become more equitable across the board, cast artists with disabilities. Do not cast a non-disabled actor in a disabled role unless you make it a policy of working with many different artists and also are casting artists with disabilities in the same play perhaps in non-disabled roles. Often a non-disabled actor will be seen to be playing the disability and its technicalities, not the character. If you aren't mixing it up like that though, please cast disabled artists in disabled roles. Reflect reality.

So, if artists need to be recruited what is it that you need to attract them? ADA compliance helps in your theatre space and most theatre spaces have some ADA compliance (if they do not and you cannot make the adjustments to make them accessible then you need to work in another space) you should be able to offer large print scripts, with a minimum eighteen to twenty point font size, and other items (many of which are dependent upon the actors you are seeking and you can find them listed on the companion website), wheelchair ramps, and honest discussion and 'disability consciousness' training of your staff.

Disability consciousness impels and is informed by the social movement actions that are happening within the disability world and culture. Having a staff aware of the disabled norms and political movements and social issues not only makes them more well-rounded as people, but allows them to truly understand and work with those who dwell within that culture. Simple things that you might think are obvious, such as do not refer to a person as their disability. (I once had a casting director tell me he needed a 'wheelchair' for his television show. Restraining myself I looked him square in the eye and said calmly, "You mean you would like to find an actor in a wheelchair? Or do you want a wheelchair yourself because you may be in it?" He was on his own after that, and oddly his casting office closed within the year.) Disabled people are not their disabilities. There are two kinds of barriers to disabled artists, human and physical. Do not let your staff, teachers, fellow cast, students or board members become human barriers.

Being ADA compliant and dealing with physical barriers, by the way, does not mean "we have an elevator." It does not stop with that. It means how do they get in the elevator, can they turn their chair in the elevator, and once they get out of the elevator do the hallways support their wheelchair or are they too narrow? Can a wheelchair make full turns to find rooms or offices? If so, can they enter the actual office or is the doorway too narrow? Can they enter the restroom (and there really should be at least one fully accessible restroom in every building in the USA) and once in the restroom can they even get into the stall? Are there grab bars in the stall? Is there room to get out of the wheelchair in the stall? Can they turn around in the hallway or must they back all the way out and into the elevator?

Are there automatic doors in the building? Do the curbs to the building have cuts so the wheelchair users can wheel themselves up? Can they even find a place to park if they drive in? Can a blind person using a cane (or blind stick as they call them) navigate the hallways? Are there no carpets or tripping obstacles? Can they even open the front door and go through? (There should be eighteen inches of clear wall space on the pull side of the door, next to the handle.) Even a great app like 'WheelMate' (which can give some accessible information to wheelchair users) can only take into account so much. You or your theatre or university should be doing the rest.

Do a check for braille text in the main elevator at least if you are expecting blind actors, as well as audible crosswalk indicators and audible elevator door opening/closing and floor indicators as well. It is not enough to ever simply have an elevator. If there are existing ramps in the building or around the stage or rehearsal rooms, are they non-slip? They should be. If the ramps are longer than six feet they should have railings on both sides. Disabled artists need to feel safe in the space, in the process and in their trust and work with you, safer than non-disabled actors need to feel. Another point about ramps is that they are not only needed for folks in wheelchairs. We have had elderly patrons, young kids, delivery men and just folks with sprained ankles or bad knees be delighted when we have ramps instead of stairs.

Every so often I encounter an artist who, because of a degenerative disease, or a TBI may feel that they are on a kind of timeline. They may rush into auditions and rehearsals and have a self-imposed stress level. They may feel that they only have so many years left on their feet, or with the use of their hands or with nimbleness of speech or so forth. With many degenerative illnesses the same actor may not be able to do the same things in five or ten years (and many times they can, you never know). It helps if you are aware of this with your artists so that you can work with them to relax and embrace and enjoy what they can do now and they can begin to be free to create even if they do feel rushed for time. Neither they nor you know what time is to be had, so when those cases arise work with them to embrace the now.

Case Study 4: Dionysus Theatre in Houston, Texas

Deborah Nowinski, Artistic Director

History

In 2006 Dionysus Theatre, founded in 1998, produced *The Voice of The Prairie* by John Olive. The play features the leading role being played by a woman who is blind. Usually this is played, both younger and older, by one actress, however we at Dionysus Theatre wanted to spread the work around and cast two different actors. Or we tried to. We had cast a wonderful actress, Marquia Banks, who is blind, in the older role and the search was on for a younger actress to play this potentially life-changing role. We needed an African-American girl who was visually impaired. Dionysus being a well-known company helped, but sometimes a very specific need involving age, racial makeup and disability can test the mettle of any company.

Plan

We went through organizations, we networked and we sent work out to schools that worked with students who were blind. It started to look, after a month of intensive searching, like a non-starter. What could we do? What would you do?

See Chapter 16 for further details of this case study.

Chapter Action: Write an Audition Ad

(A template is on the companion website.)

Remember to create an ad where you ask for what you want – are you casting an artist with a specific disability in a role? Have you been on the lookout for a disabled artist of color or gender? Be very specific and always remember what your capacity is as a theatre to support both off- and onstage. Tell them what you can offer – stipend, Access-a-Ride or something similar during performances, childcare if needed? Explain your parameters (time, commitment, location) and be very specific. Will they be needed at every rehearsal or can you augment their schedule?

5

AUDITIONS AND CALLBACKS

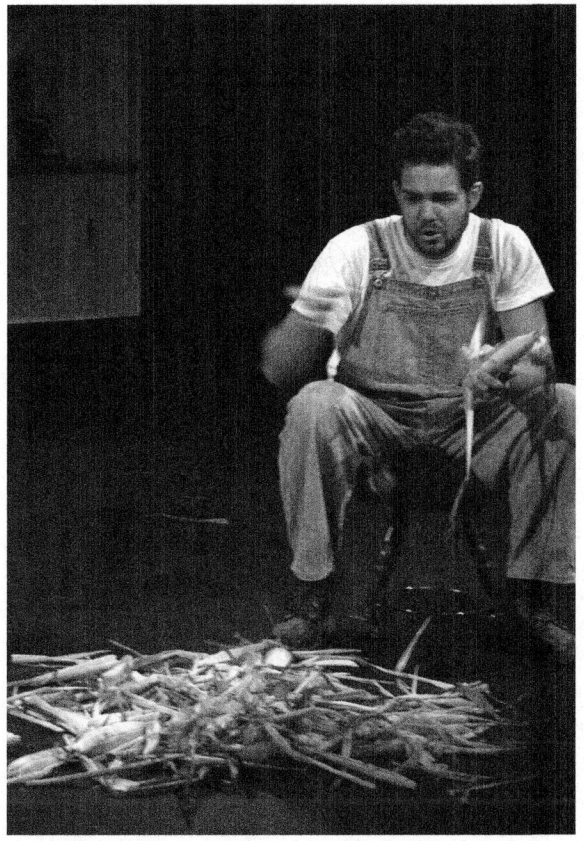

Figure 5.1   Dax (Darren Fudenske) in *Buried Child* by Sam Shepard, 2006.
(Photograph courtesy of Nicu's Spoon Theater Company.)

The biggest problem about the casting issue is that the casting issue is nowhere near the biggest problem. Casting is the window dressing. Until we look at the system as a whole and have disabled artists in positions which afford them the opportunity to make root-level changes (they) are nothing more than tokens.

Brad Rothbart, American Theatre Magazine, October 2015, *Once More Unto the Breach: An Anatomized Philippic Regarding the Relationship of Disability to the Contemporary American Theatre*

Your auditions, whether as a theatre company or as an academic institution looking for new theatre students, are only as good as your preparation for them. To ensure your sanity and theirs always give every artist an appointment time so they know they are respected and you know you have time to spend with them. Do not ever do general open calls with artists with disabilities. You do not want a room filled with wheelchairs, crutches, blind sticks and so forth. It is a hazard and you (and they) need calm. That will only increase stress for everyone. Lead the way by planning the audition well and it will serve you, and them, well.

As I do actively recruit and invite artists in I know almost all of them via email or Skype or through having seen or met them somewhere and thus by the time we meet we do feel as if we know each other, at least a little bit. I already may have ideas in my brain of ways we could cast them or cross-disability cast various performers, although I inevitably look forward to the artist's own strengths to give me new ideas. I am not a big believer, as a director or producer, that you must be cruel and break actors down and make them fear you in order to teach or direct. Love makes miracles, so I touch them and love them and I listen to them. I am not saying you should do this, but I do. Every now and again, heartbreakingly, I have been told that I hug some actors with more love than some of their families show them. It costs you nothing to be kind and show it. Kindness equals respect. Kindness equals investment.

I am also acutely aware that many disabled artists struggle with (as many actors of color did many years ago in the 1950s and 1960s) being able to 'pass' as non-disabled artists, but then if they can pass should they do so? How much of themselves and their identity as an artist with a disability do they sacrifice in order to be cast? How then do they carry themselves around their disabled colleagues being the one who 'passes?' There is also the constant stress of passing and worrying when the ability to do that will end. This can cause enormous stress for artists which you need to see and understand. Many artists with a mental or developmental disability or a TBI may 'pass' at first glance, but they are no less a concern for you to make sure they are comfortable.

'Neuronormatives' is a newer term in the disability community, as is 'neurotypical' (both terms are traditionally used in academic writings, but have now moved into mainstream conversations both inside and outside the disability community). Both terms address those with the neurology that is standard issue, with neurodiversity as an encouraged and celebrated alternative. Those who are members of the neurodiverse community can include the aforementioned developmentally disabled, those with autism, transgendered individuals and those who have encountered neurological injury or deterioration. The neurodiverse may 'pass' in some cases (in fact, in many cases), however it is up to us as colleagues and collaborators to lessen their stress by supporting and understanding their struggles. This is important in academic circles as well, as this is yet another community that is finding its footing in social forums, gatherings, power and political activism. This is yet another segment of the disability community that is speaking up with one voice.

The trend now in casting (as more and more disabled and neurodiverse actors find work) is to cast the disabled artists who have the most immediately identifiable disabilities, wheelchair users being 'hot' right now. Being in a wheelchair is immediately identifiable as a disability, for both Broadway and for film and television as well, thus the audience does not have to think or learn anything new, no explanation is needed, and it can seem pretty straightforward to a new director in working with that actor. The Ivo Van Hove directed production of Tennessee Williams' *The Glass Menagerie* which opened on Broadway in 2017, stars Sally Field as Amanda and, after an exhaustive national search, a young actress, Madison Ferris, has been cast as Laura. Madison is an extremely talented actress and she is also in a wheelchair. Her being in a wheelchair works better than her being an amputee or having CP for two reasons. One, she is immediately identifiable as a disabled actress and two, she can then appear smaller onstage, and easily subservient, than the lead (Sally Field, who is a petite woman). Madison, I have no doubt, will be brilliant (and a new and much needed role model for young disabled actresses) and yet, I do expect that at some juncture someone will think outside that wheelchair box and explore new disability aesthetics and new mobility issues, some that may require the audience to think harder. This obvious disability and wheelchairs issue, in and of itself, sets up a hierarchy of casting within the disabled community with wheelchair users being at the apex of the most castable.

We put out widely open season calls nearly every year for disabled playwrights, who often seem to be a forgotten group, and have worked with many including Ruth Beiber (her play *To see or not to see* allowed us to work with her own life story as a young blind girl), and Raymond Luczak, a brilliant playwright who is deaf (we produced his play *Love in the Veins* which is written for two deaf actors signing in ASL, and we had two speaking actors simultaneously voice it so once again we could share it with both deaf and hearing audiences) and many others over the years. Again, recruit and ask specifically for what you are looking for. But be ready for them when they arrive.

One way to be ready for any auditioner, but in particular for actors with disabilities, is to have a trained audition monitor. In standard audition practice, monitors check in actors, manage lobby traffic, distribute audition scenes, hand out and retrieve information sheets from auditioners and help out where needed. Monitors should be well-versed in at least the basics of ASL as well as having training in sensitivity and specific helpful responses to artists who have a spectrum of disabilities.

Wheelchair etiquette is another thing that should be tackled in staff and/or cast training. The wheelchair of a cast member is not for others to play with, lean on, sit in or push whether the person is in it or not. It is, again, an extension of that person and you should no more do any of these things than you should grab another person's arm and start picking your nose with it. In addition, school your cast and staff to not give help or push the wheelchair without being asked. Non-disabled people in particular do not have an obligation or job to help any disabled person. Only help if asked to.

A word, though, about little people. Little people, or those of short stature, is the preferred term for those with dwarfism (of which achondroplasia is the most common form). This group within the disability community at large still seems to be one of the most publicly mistreated, and the fact that it seems to still be socially 'OK' and 'Politically Correct' to stare at them and treat them oddly or ignore them entirely is something that needs specific thought and a shift in thinking. They, as well as the rest of the disabled community, must be treated with respect. There are common-sense ways to do this. For me, addressing someone to their face is vitally important so often I will kneel to talk to a little person or I will suggest we both sit together so our faces are level. It is a measure of respect. Practicing respect is one of the things you and your company or university must do in order to be human, let alone work with any artists, disabled or not.

I often get asked about insurance and how much more the costs increase when working with disabled artists. There is an odd myth that we must have to have millions of dollars of insurance. This is yet another myth grown up out of not having enough information. We have the same standard insurances we have always had for our shows (different, of course, if your shows tour or move to a bigger venue or cross a state line) and have always insured not only all our artists, but also all our audiences with the usual insurance that any company or theatre space should have. We have *never* incurred additional insurance costs because we work with artists with disabilities. This is yet another myth.

You and your staff, however, do have the responsibility to not only dispel myths, but to be ready for artists by double-checking all accessibility which again includes restrooms and halls, not just the elevator. Depending upon who you will be seeing at your audition and what they may need (and you should put yourself in the place of every actor whom you will see, and think "What can we do to make your audition a comfortable one?") you also should or could provide braille (with some advance notice) or large print scenes and a volunteer or audition monitor who can assist (they may run lines or they may stand behind a blind actor and calmly feed them lines as they audition), as well try to have no scented perfumes or heavy smells around as this can trigger various disabilities. There are various computer programs (and apps like VIA) that are also useful that speak to the actor who is blind via his or her iPad or headphones. You can allow artists access to the audition room for a bit ahead of time if needed and/or have a second quiet room for centering. For your disabled staff you can focus on more ergonomic workplaces if you have a production office.

Music stands are also very helpful for auditions as deaf performers – or performers with one arm or hand/arm mobility issues – who are auditioning can use them so they can still see the text but have (in the case of deaf actors) both hands free to sign or relax as they need to. Invest in three or so music stands now as they will be endlessly useful. You can provide music and acoustic checks if needed for singing auditions. Have an ASL interpreter if needed, and have the ability to lower lights in the room if needed.

Emailing audition scenes to actors way ahead of time for an audition is a general good bet for all artists, but especially for any translation into braille readers for the blind or audio files they can listen to. Lastly give the entire day *time*, give the actors auditioning time and give them time to meet each other as well. Give yourself time to be surprised and enjoy them. I still remember a lovely young actor coming in and nailing an audition for Jem in *To Kill a Mockingbird*. (He thought outside the box as an actor and I immediately wanted to work with him.) But, I also gave myself the time in the audition to really see him, enjoy him and then be crazy about him. I was not so overwhelmed that I missed him in the stress of that day. Now, he runs his own company in New York City which develops disabled playwrights (who easily produce the most challenging and imaginative and honest work in the US today).

I know that this may seem overwhelming, just thinking about large print audition scenes to help at auditions and also wheelchair access, but trust me it is not hard once you just pick one thing and start with that. Start with something you know you can do – do you have an ASL interpreter whom you know? Start with hiring a deaf actor. Just start.

Many actors (both disabled and non-disabled) love working with my company and others like it because it gives them the chance to work with other artists with disabilities that they do not yet know from the disabled community. Just because two people are disabled does not mean they automatically know each other or every other disabled person in the world. Simply because an artist has MS doesn't mean they know or understand another artist who may have MS, and it certainly doesn't mean they would immediately understand an artist who is blind or is an amputee. *Everyone* learns about each other by working together toward a common goal, the production.

A special note for the artists with disabilities who are auditioning. You have the right to be in accessible spaces, to be assisted in any way you need. I want you to have every aspect of what you need so that you are able to give me the best audition you can. However, if you are in a situation where your needs are not being met, or are being ignored entirely, or you are being shut down you have the right to speak up and educate as to what is needed. Even if you are at a union audition where things should be more organized and you realize you cannot access the stage to audition, you must speak up. Do not leave the audition as if it is your failing, it is not. Unfortunately sometimes you must be a teacher.

In 2002 we held auditions for *To Kill a Mockingbird* and actively asked for disabled artists to audition. This was still early in our history so we had to actively find folks. I had many young men audition for the role of Jem, but at one point this young fellow (previously mentioned) named Gregg Mozgala came in and blew us all away with his very physical audition, fearless and fully appropriate for Jem who is in that place between teen and young man. I was pretty sure Gregg had CP and yet he had given the most physically realized audition I had seen and I loved the idea and spirit behind that. Of course I cast him, and within the context of that play he brought a weight to lines the audience heard anew. During the court scene, for instance, when Jem finally sees Tom Robinson and exclaims, "He's a cripple!" it meant something new and important coming from a disabled actor. In many plays with us in following years, as well as letting us do his own play *Spaz* in our 2005 reading series, Gregg became a company member and now many years later he has a company himself, the Apothetae, which develops disabled playwrights, and he acts and dances and advocates and writes and makes the world an infinitely better, more creative and more interesting place. I am lucky to know him.

Before you cast your show (at about the time you are deciding callbacks) you should know if you will be using union or non-union performers, or both. Dealing with the unions (AEA is the stage union) and their contracts do not become any more complicated because you have disabled artists in your cast. AEA does not require any more technical things for artists with disabilities working on a show. The only thing you may want to deal with is special agreements for things that are filmed.

I've mentioned that in 2013 a documentary crew followed our company for about eight months through audition and show preparation, rehearsals and full performances of *The Cherry Orchard*. The finished documentary, *Two and Twenty Troubles* (directed by Victor Ilyukhin), was completed because of the kind cooperation of AEA in New York City who allowed the special filming of both rehearsals and performances for the documentary. It has since gone on to be in many festivals and the link to it is in the Resources section at the back of this book.

Since we are on the subject of AEA contracts, also keep in mind whether you have plans for your show to tour. If you do, then you should meet with each and every disabled artist after they are cast and see what they will need in order to be comfortable on the road. For some there is nothing extra, but for others they may need a wheelchair accessible hotel room with everything set at a lower level for them, or a room with everything in braille. If you all do not leave the state but instead drive around town in a bus to local schools and tour that way then you still need to see what everyone needs.

In thinking of what people need, sometimes I have found that what they and I both need is an audition that *is not* an audition. In 2015 we co-produced *Richard III* with the New York City company Identity Theater. About twenty-five actors who were new to the company were called, recruited and recommended to audition for roles alongside the company members. When they got to the audition I surprised them by not wanting to see their prepared monologues or giving them scenes. All we did was just sit and talk, like people, about them, their art, their life, what they thought about the play. I have sat through millions of auditions in my life and by now I know talent when it walks in the door. I do not need to see a monologue that they have been doing for years and all the patterns, breathing and emotions have been set in it (this tells me nothing about them). I want to see them revealed.

What I do not know in an audition is who this person is, truly is, and how we can create art together. If you then create a safe space you may find that they feel so safe that you do discuss cochlear implants and the controversy around them, or those who persist in treating autism or alopecia as diseases of the mind that are not real. With autism on the rise, and appearing in one out of eighty-eight births, it is something that must be accepted and discussed. If we talk about it at an audition that is all okay in my book. You are seeing disabled actors so let the auditions be what they need to be.

For example, that day for *Richard III* we saw a young actor named Ian Gregory Hill. He was thrilled not to have to do a monologue and to actually just get to sit and talk to someone. As we talked he discussed his autism and the fact that ASL was actually his first language, as his family had thought he was deaf for the first few years of his life. I already knew in my head by then that I was definitely casting him in the show, but his saying that immediately made me see a scene full blown in my head. He ended up playing a few roles in *Richard III* for us, but my favorite one and a real show-stopping moment was when he played Tyrell (who murders the young princes) as a deaf man, so he signed and softly spoke the role. When Tyrell has his speech about the deaths of the princes we orchestrated the music, lights and his own movement and signing to all represent the sadness he felt for carrying this out. To this day people mention this scene to me and how affecting it was, and I literally 'saw' it happen in my mind's eye during our first audition meeting by using information which was true to life about that specific artist. Ian is now union and touring with shows and working like mad, so our show was a great place for him to be seen and to show off his talent both verbally and with ASL.

A special note if you have a touring company going out, as some shows you may want to tour, make sure your stage manager makes a note as to all the needed medicines of the cast (*all* the cast, not just those with disabilities), prescription numbers and doctors' telephone numbers. It doesn't help to run out of medicines in the middle of Peoria.

Will your show end up going from an off-off Broadway (or the equivalent where you are) run and then move to an Off-Broadway contracted run or a larger venue? We had one that did and more than a few actors were able to get their union cards because of it. Things like this are very exciting, but you still have to make sure you walk the new stage with the blind actor and pace it all out carefully and ensure the cues are reset for all who need them. Do not let a show's success or any personal successes, or even other people's perception of the success ("Hey that is so great, let's go celebrate, you do not need to do things at the theatre!") distract you from any artists' needs.

How do we be aware of artists' needs in letting actors know they are cast or called back? In your auditions you should create an audition sheet which is handed to each prospective artist that gets all the information you need from them (contact information, their address and all numbers and emails and TTY/TDD information, their preferred method of contact – this is very important, their conflicts during planned rehearsal dates and any other information; a template is on the companion website). Make sure everyone fills this out. Have someone assist them if needed, but get this information from everyone.

Callbacks are about the same as auditions, but you can add even one more reader for practice with callback scenes. There is a great company (Phamaly Theatre, founded in 1989, and to my mind the role model for any theatre thinking to embrace inclusive casting) in Denver who has 'Social Stories' on their website for autistic and developmentally disabled individuals. The social story is a pictorial tour of what to expect at auditions and callbacks, what things look like, what color the door they go in may be, where they are going to go. Things like this are why Phamaly is one of the top most caring, dynamic and inclusive theatres in the US.

Then after callbacks we sit down and cast. We have never not cast someone because of a disability. Ever. We cast according to the best person or the most interesting energy in the role (keeping in mind that we already have a vision for the show in our heads). After this I have my stage manager either email or call each artist we are calling back depending upon their preferred method of contact. We do the same with our final casting of the show as well. I, in addition, always email the actors who are *not* cast to thank them for their audition, to tell them I understand that their time is precious and I am grateful they spent it with us and to ask them to *please* return and audition for us again. And I do mean it. And we do see them auditioning for us again. Then we see if they accept the role or roles we cast them in, as sometimes our casting even surprises them (in a good way).

Every now and then I may encounter an artist with a disability who doesn't want to accept a role that they may feel is traditionally cast as a pitiable disabled role (Laura in *The Glass Menagerie* comes to mind, and there will be more on this role later). Then it becomes my job to let them see that ninety-nine percent of the time the past casting of the role has been with non-disabled artists and it is about time a disabled actor performed the role and made new discoveries and new interpretations. I urge them to throw out old notions, prejudices and ideas and to approach the role as if they have never seen it before and thankfully this usually works.

In 2008 I asked a young actress/model/writer named Margaret Baker to work with us on a new play we had been developing for two years, *A Kite Cut Loose in the Middle of the Sky* by David Greenberg. I asked her to play a few roles, one non-disabled and one with a disability that in *no way* resembled hers. Margaret has alopecia universalis and began to lose her hair at about six years old. In addition to the alopecia and the hardship that brought, there were many other things in her life that made it tough. She had a tough childhood and had survived and I had already known her about two or three years and both adored and respected her. I asked her to play a woman who had lost both arms completely and then both legs below the knee. It was a tough, mouthy, highly sexually charged role and Margaret jumped in with both feet and was great. She later commented on what a relaxing and wonderful thing it had been to play someone without alopecia, to be able to just really get into another disability's head and learn some new things and new angles of 'disability' that had not been on her radar before. The bonus of playing a disabled role that was sexualized was even better.

Case Study 5: Can an Actor Who Is Deaf Speak? Nicu's Spoon Theater, New York City

History

In 2006 we were in pre-production (we plan our shows six months or more in advance) for *Buried Child* by Sam Shepard, and as I was directing I was reading and rereading the text and it came to me that there was a character in the play who had very few lines, and seemed to always have people repeat what he just said and then respond. ("Where did you get that?" "Picked it." "Picked it, where?" "Out back." "Out back?") And so forth. A great deal of repetition, as well as many times where other characters said, "What?" repeatedly, forcing the character of Tilden to repeat himself. As I looked more deeply at this role, which had been traditionally treated as if he had some level of developmental or intellectual disability or was simply burned out, it came to me that perhaps it could be played by a deaf actor. But not a deaf actor signing, a deaf actor speaking – fully speaking.

Why speaking? Because it was a play about secrets and denial and lies that families tell that have repercussions into generations. A play about a family in denial about who they are and things they have done to their children and each other. In giving the play a new aspect, that a son had been born deaf and mute but had not been acknowledged as such nor given any kind of ASL or Deaf culture access, I felt we could enhance this dark and beautiful piece even more. Also, being a very well-known play, it gave us a great opportunity to shake up 'set in stone' notions about how to do it. There was nothing in our rights agreement that said we could not cast like this, as the deaf actor would be fully verbalizing the role, so we did.

I had at the time recently audited a show for the New York State Council on the Arts at the New York Deaf Theatre based in Brooklyn, and had been overwhelmed by a talented young actor named Darren Fudenske (Dax for short). He was the perfect actor for this role in *Buried Child*, but how could I convince him to break down some societal, cultural (Deaf culture is a very strong culture) and even personal and familial barriers and speak an entire role for a month of rehearsals and a three-week run and not sign at all onstage?

Plan

I approached him with the idea as well as who I was and what my company did. Luckily he knew of us and we began the first of many conversations and I know he did some *very* deep soul searching. He might get flack from the Deaf community for speaking when he was a deaf actor. He might get flack from the hearing community for speaking. We both might get tarred and feathered. Uniquely, he came from an entirely deaf family and who knows what they may have thought? Dax said later in a *New York Times* interview:

> It's very hard. I have to keep in my head who I am. I'm always using my hands. I love to use my hands. That's my first language. But at the same time I'm an actor so I have to separate the two.
>
> *NY Times Arts & Leisure*, October 15, 2006
> 'An Actor Uses His Second Language: Speech'
> by Steven McElroy

To this day I do not know why Dax finally agreed to do it. Perhaps because we had just created a new theatre performance style the year before called co-playing and had presented *Stumps* by Mark Medoff with a half-signing and half-speaking cast. Some incredibly talented deaf actors had worked with us on that, and Dax knew them from the Deaf community and perhaps that is why he said yes. But he said yes. So, now you have a deaf actor who has never really spoken in life, let alone onstage before and you have cast him in a speaking role. What is your step-by-step checklist to getting him to performance? Certainly, working with him to produce sound, enunciate, and so forth, but think of him and the cast and make a step-by-step process list of what you would do for this case study.

See Chapter 16 for further details of this case study.

Chapter Action: Make an Audition or Callback Checklist

(Many ideas and helpful suggestions about how to accommodate, plan for, schedule and structure can be found on the companion website.)

A last note, whether in audition or callbacks, is to keep your groupings small so you can always deal with individuals. This is something I do even with non-disabled actors. Crowds at callbacks are problematic normally anyway, but for an autistic individual or someone in a wheelchair they can become nerve-racking. For yourself as well, you do yourself and your production a disservice if you do not have the space to make time to 'see,' really see, each of the auditioners as human beings and artists. I do not conduct auditions where the actor leaves and I know nothing about them. I want to see the person under the artist.

6

REHEARSALS

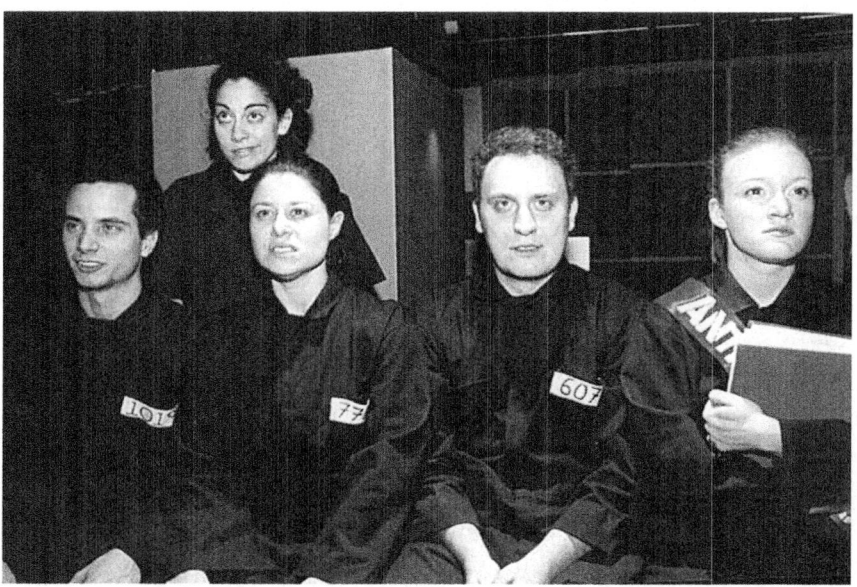

Figure 6.1 George Orwell's *1984* adapted by Robert Owens, Wilton E. Hall, Jr. and William A. Miles, Jr., 2003. L to R Gregg Mozgala, Jennifer Stokes, Mary Holmstrom, Daniel Rappaport and Natalie Blair. (Photograph courtesy of Nicu's Spoon Theater Company.)

Since 2001, Barton-Farcas's theater company, Nicu's Spoon, has worked to de-objectify its diverse base of performers to create a dynamic and proficient group of artists. With a proven commitment to working for social change in theater by populating it—both onstage and backstage—with performers of all shapes, sizes, colors, ages, and abilities, Nicu's Spoon has produced risky and thought-provoking productions, earning kudos from both audiences and critics.

OffOffOnline, Amy Krivohlavek, 2007

So, you have finally cast your show. You have contacted all your new actors and have them headed in for your first full cast meeting and read-through. Now you should be beginning the process of investing in knowing them and their needs as individual artists, so before your first full meet as a cast have a meeting with your immediate production staff, which means your stage manager and any ASMs and/or production assistants and interns. Talk about each actor and any issues that need keeping an eye on so you are all on the same page. You may have artists or designers with multiple and/or differing disabilities (i.e. an actor who is intellectually disabled and is also blind or a designer who is deaf and also has ADHD and CP) and, again although they are not treated with any kid gloves or special treatment, the information simply needs to be understood by the staff. Then eat pizza! In theatre, pizza is a great bonding mechanism. For my company not only is it the literal eating together, but it also can become a shared experience between an artist who is disabled and one who is not (and has never worked with one who is) or one who is gay and one who is a straight eighty year old. Silly as it sounds, many an unusual and long-term friendship has begun in our company simply by eating pizza together.

Eating together at the outset also sets the stage for the involvement of all of the senses in our work. We eat as we listen, as we watch each other, as we laugh and feel and reach out and touch each other. If one or more of us is minus one of these senses (or two) then the simultaneous involvement of these senses all together, as a shared group, not only bonds us but makes those who are not minus a sensory input bond with and get on board with those who are different. As we work with both disabled and non-disabled artists of every color, age, gender and gender spectrum expression, religion and nationality, things like this, simple eating together, become much more than a meal at a first rehearsal. There is nothing like breaking bread to start a cast off right. Eating together is an ancient rite, breaking bread brings us together as a tribe.

One of the things my company has done over the years when needed is to assist both the disabled and non-disabled artists alike with childcare, as we found that particularly for women and single parents this was one of the additional barriers to returning to the arts. We have been able to have extra interns trade off on the nights kids are there (as we have artists bring them to our theatre or rehearsal space) and help with childcare while the parent is rehearsing. Many disabled people are parents and this has been another way we can not only support them, but let them be assured that their kids are well and safe because they can see them in the lobby during breaks. Another thing we have done, in casts of young women, disabled and non-disabled, is made sure they were escorted to their car, cab, Access-a-Ride or to the bus and subway. These things, again, are examples of things that can be done for low to no cost and it means the world to your artists.

As you have the first full cast/staff meeting and read-through, continue the support you began with and add orientation for all of them to the room and building you will be rehearsing in. Disability status changes with the environment, so make sure you have an environment where every single performer has access and space. Then you all start from a place of full ability and equity. If you all start from a place of full ability, then you can begin to discover the things that keep people from each other and away from creating art. Even 'flaws' in a body can become the entry points into new ideas, performance moments or actions. Thus there becomes a freedom in the disabled body that there may never be in a non-disabled one. Each body has something to say, statements to make and stories to tell and each artist benefits from being with others and being a part of something greater.

Be sure to adhere to solid break times – you must anyway if you have any union actors – but especially for actors who are disabled (or elderly or very young) having set break times is a great policy. Have everyone introduce themselves and introduce any facilitators as well (ASL interpreters or even caregivers for artists who may be present at rehearsal). Try to go around the room and let each of your actors and staff say a bit about themselves. (I always try to have the designers also present at the first read-through.) If your company has a PR representative, they should be invited to first read-throughs or a few rehearsals. Make time for the artists and staff and after that read the play (even if you have to speed through the second act because you run out of time; connections between people are the primary focus for the first read-through).

I have already named a few things you should talk about in your first cast meeting, but there is also a checklist on the companion website (www.routledge.com/cw/barton-farcas) which can act as a template that you can then add or subtract from. In your first cast meet and read-through always opt for being more informative as opposed to less. Information truly is power.

The actors and I do talk in further rehearsals about their role development and about how they feel about being what and who they are in the play, about how it is to be deaf, autistic, a little person in life, etc. and how that may or may not inform their work on the role. However, we talk about it only if it is important or if it comes up. If they are cast in a role with a disability they do not have, then we talk about that and work together on it. Most of the time they are simply cast for who they are and then the role (no matter what the classical depiction of it has been in the past) has the same disability as them forevermore.

As you leave your first read-through behind and enter your formal rehearsals, keep in mind generally the sooner you can block the better. Especially for the complicated blocking sequences when you have perhaps the whole cast onstage. We also have major props and any weapons in our rehearsals sooner as opposed to later. Specialty props we often have from the very first blocking rehearsal. We block immediately in rehearsals (even if it ends up being totally different in final performances, as it often is) as for many disabled artists, and a great many non-disabled artists, knowing where they are and where they need to be in the space is the first priority. Often actors cannot learn lines unless they know where they are physically, so we block as soon as we enter rehearsals.

The early physicality of blocking also impacts the neuroplasticity of the brain and body for those with disabilities. The more repetition and challenge they are handed, and the earlier the better, the more it encourages cortical excitability and stimulation. The idea that the brain is plastic and can be constantly changing and impacted to change at any age is a concept that is gaining ground in the scientific community, however those who work within the disabled community and in theatre have known this for years. The nervous system can be constantly and consistently challenged and given greater work to do and all bodies, even (and sometimes especially) disabled ones, will rise to the occasion and adapt. The outward confidence and personal power that comes with these challenges and changes is equally important for the artist or designer with a disability.

To the above rehearsals and blocking add in any needed augmented scheduling, perhaps having to stagger rehearsal scenes for certain actors only on the few nights in a week that they have solid transportation into the theatre. Use the artists according to their schedule and transportation and travel ability. Keep in mind that often disabled people are in quite inequitable money situations if they are employed (perhaps making much less in a lower paying job as employers who should be hiring them often are not) and it may be more difficult for them to not only physically get to and from rehearsal, but also to foot the bill in emergencies. We have often had emergency funds for each project where an actor who is stuck and really must be in rehearsal can call a taxi or car service and we reimburse them for it. Things like this are part of a well-thought-out and ongoing commitment to fully inclusive casting.

Always make certain there are notes in the stage manager's and ASM's production books regarding medications or cast needs (we have learned to *always* have an ASM – or even two – if your cast is above fourteen actors). Additionally, services such as Access-A-Ride or others in your city which transport wheelchair users and artists with mobility issues should be on a call list which your stage manager has at all times. An added tip is that if you have a board member or community donor then ask them to foot the bill for transportation needs for one show for your artists with disabilities, then you have your private van or ride provider paid for.

As you move into more complicated work if needed (singing, dancing, physically intimate scenes, fight choreography) be aware that not only should production staff write it all out by hand but if you can also take pictures or record musical numbers, fight sequences or complicated staging do so for reference online for the cast. (We would put all fight or dance choreography on a private YouTube channel with only the actors being able to log on and watch it.) People learn in different ways, so some artists may benefit from the fight sequences being written out, while others may need to see them visually and watch them repeatedly. You also, of course, run them at every rehearsal where applicable. I also treat any physically intimate scenes (makeouts, sexual moments or the like) as I do fight scenes. We choreograph them in detail and do it early in the process so the actors have more time to be physically comfortable with each other. If need be, have the actors sit with the stage manager before a rehearsal and review every bit of staging or blocking as much as they need to. We have also had the stage managers or ASMs write down blocking and send it by email to certain actors who perhaps have no ability to write it out for themselves. The key is approaching the needs from all angles and then filling in the blanks as needed.

Often as you work with actors you will ask them to do things nobody has ever asked them to do before. In 2011 we presented a wonderful short story by author John Langan, *How the Day Runs Down* (like *Our Town* by Thornton Wilder, but with zombies), as a play. Katie Labahn, now a Las Vegas based actress/playwright and a long-time company member (and also the owner/user of an awesome manual wheelchair which looked right out of some marathon race), was in the show and I asked her how she might feel if we started the show with her, but not staying in the wheelchair as she had always performed with us. My idea was that the audience would think she was a dead body when they entered, but then she would reanimate, slide out of the wheelchair and crawl herself across the stage. I had known her for many years and had never asked her to get out of the chair before and as I did ask her my brain went, "Yikes! Should I have asked differently? Or not at all?" She sat for a second and then said, "Yeah, I love that idea! How awesome!" and promptly popped herself out of the chair and commenced dragging herself around and delighting in freaking the cast out. She is a gloriously terrific gal and her sweetness hides her innate gutsy-as-heck attitude, but in retrospect I also know now that she knew she was safe, respected and that if she said "No" I would say, "Ok, no worries, here's another idea."

I have also learned to always have understudies if you have any precarious health issues with a main artist and always have a Plan B set up. I have had artists have to leave productions because of surgeries or health issues, however that is never in my mind when I cast them and offer roles. Just as with non-disabled artists there is no way to predict who will or will not have issues, so put it out of your mind when casting.

Each artist (even the non-disabled, I have found) has their own personal challenge for themselves and for you. There is also a pointed difference in an artist born with a disability and someone who is newly (within the past three years) disabled. There is a rawness with someone newly disabled, as they are not quite 'at home' in the disability yet, as well as many possible further physical complications that someone who was born dealing with a disability may not have. For a newer disabled person the accident, injury, impairment happened all at once – however, it takes years to 'be' disabled. The author Simi Linton talks about 'becoming disabled' years after the accident that changed her body. Stress from these traumatic events and even repeated surgeries can lead to PTSD. PTSD has many symptoms and may include mood swings, flashbacks and uncontrollable emotions. Very little study has been done on PTSD in people with both physical and mental disabilities, however it certainly does exist. Moreover, from children on up, those with disabilities suffering with PTSD can be helped. Just being aware of this and being open to any conversations that may be needed and being fully supportive of each artist's physical and emotional journey is a good place to start.

Play (as in let's play!) is vitally important in rehearsal. Musical games for the deaf and hearing in the cast (turn the music UP and everyone feel the vibrations!), dancing with the blind (stand facing them or stand behind them and teach them the steps!), non-deaf people signing in ASL (we always learn the dirty signs first), rehearsals for us are for continually exploring the crossover of boundaries and the world of each disability and inviting each artist to begin doing what they normally do not do. In our first co-played production, *Stumps* (and in a few subsequent productions), we had a few rehearsals where I had the hearing actors wear earplugs so they really had to work hard to communicate and they got a small taste of their co-playing counterparts' lives. In no way did it compare to them being deaf, but it made them feel closer to understanding their deaf co-player and a place of connection like that is never a bad thing. Often for mental and developmental disabilities the response to games, music and general silliness is the best warm up you can do. Once they get the sillies and dancing out the artists are usually much more able to focus on blocking or lines. For those artists with TBI, mental or developmental issues, art, jobs, work and activity and performance is therapy. Even the most extreme TBI injuries can be helped with performance, although the later perceptions of that performance can sometimes alter themselves within the damaged brain. For those artists with no disabilities at all performance is also therapy. Understand that all of us, disabled or not, sometimes need to get 'jiggy' and get the physical wacky out of ourselves so then we can settle down and attend to the 'serious' making of art. I have also, on one occasion, had an actor break down and cry after dancing as he said he felt something, 'release and let go' and he then moved into rehearsals with a new sense of purpose. Don't underestimate the power of play and movement.

In 2015, our fifteenth season, my company co-produced *Richard III* (we did it in 2007 and again in 2015), and I directed in 2015 as well. For this new world of the play our entire society was a disabled one, everyone around Richard is disabled, the world is geared to the disabled and he is 'perfect' and non-disabled. Every notion about the play and that world was to be turned on its head. For example, Richmond (normally portrayed as a young strapping fellow who gives great speeches and then kills Richard III) as directed by me, is petite and an epileptic and after a few petit mal seizures in the play has a final grand mal seizure onstage in the middle of his well-known speech before fighting Richard (and how would I know what that grand mal seizure looks like? Harken ye back to Case Study 1!). But this seizure was treated as *normal* and even thought to be a gift from God in that world. We thus have many new ways to now illuminate that text onstage as we work through the play. A world where all parking spaces are for the handicapped! A world where a wheelchair moves into every single building without a second thought, where everything has braille on it, every crosslight beeps, where only those with disabilities are in power and hold jobs of high position. Where only the disabled go to college. We now see Richard III as someone who loathes himself because he is *not* disabled and wishes to be disabled so that he can be accepted. Shake things up and dare to make the audience think.

We then find many notions can be turned on their heads, such as our making *Richard III* (with a dozen varying disabilities in the cast) a *very* physical production where we sat the audience on the flat stage and had the actors performing around them on three sides and up and down on the sets of high risers that made up the 'audience area.' In the show we had crutches and sticks and props and weapons and artists in wheelchairs, both in and out of the wheelchairs, artists with prosthetics working both with and without them (and again this type of artistic trust only comes from support and true caring), a variety of sizes of people and an enormous number of fights, sexuality and physicality which most of the audience found very unexpected in their standardized thoughts about a heavily disabled cast.

The actors loved it, as for many of them (and for many artists in our production history) it is the first time they have ever gotten to do serious stage combat, handle a weapon or dance or be in physically intimate scenes or any hyper-involved kinetic movement process onstage. This type of theatre frees both the audience's ingrained perceptions of what the play should be, and the audience members' ingrained ideas about what disabled artists are capable of. The artists' notions of what they can physically and emotionally do both onstage and in real life are explored then and grow as well. Over the years many artists who work with us go on to found their own companies (I will note those in the Resources section) and others have gone on to produce their own web series, get agents, do films, move to union jobs and get union cards, go skydiving and jump into things they tell me they might not have done before working with us. This is the theatrical legacy we want to leave because these artists make the world a richer place for doing these things. They inform the world we all live in. This is the human legacy we want to leave because it is right and fair and makes the world a much richer place.

I have learned also that sometimes the physical and most obvious parts of being disabled are often the easiest for the disabled artists to deal with. I was at an audience talk back in 2015 after the *Two and Twenty Troubles* documentary screening about my company and a very unaware audience member demanded of an actress why she had to drop out of a project if her prosthetic leg gave her problems. "Couldn't you just take the leg off and do the play anyway and not have the stump be hurt? Then you could have your cake and eat it too." He snapped angrily at her with an anger the non-disabled sometimes reserve for things they do not understand.

What he didn't understand was the emotional and mental injury that comes with the new disability (and this was a fairly recently disabled person he was addressing). He had an odd notion that for a newly disabled person his unrealistic idea of, "Well, why do you not just take off the leg?" was easy for her. In reality it is a very private thing, it is your body, and to whip your prosthetic leg off can be akin for some to stripping naked in front of an audience. It is a very intimate issue, having a part of yourself not match the status quo and often people can forget that the physical is only a part of the disability. Many times the pain and healing of the mind is what may be neglected in traditional physical therapy and that is what I believe that art heals.

Case Study 6: Snow White *and* Richard III, Nicu's Spoon Theater, New York City

History

Rachel Handler is an energized and gorgeous young singer, actress and dancer. She first worked with my company in 2012 when she walked into an audition and nailed it, nabbing the lead in *Snow White and Rose Red*. There was no doubt she was Snow White and it is rare that I am that impressed. She was cast and did the show with us and I came to know her as just a hard working, talented beyond belief, genuinely good and caring person and actress. After the show was over I did something I rarely do with actors. I sat down with her and told her how very talented I really believed she was and that she had something different, something shiny and special that tons of the young, eager kids in New York City do not have. She was a true triple threat. I told her not to give up, no matter what. Mark my words, you *will* see this kid on Broadway one day. I believed it with all my heart then and I still do to this very day.

About three months after she did that show she was in an ungodly freak car accident on her way to an audition and lost her left leg from the knee down. Her life, family, career and relationships all changed in an instant. I told her in the midst of her recovery thank god she had worked with us, as I was then able to connect her up to some amazing artistic ladies (the wonderful actress/writer/singer/advocate Anita Hollander is one, and if you do not know her work – look her up! The talent, oy!) who had been where Rachel was now in her disability journey and who could help her and bolster her and understand her in ways that I knew I could not.

In her first three years of recovery I offered Rachel numerous roles, some of which she turned down because of transportation, further surgeries or other issues and some of which she accepted and then had to pull out of. At one point someone asked me, "Why do you keep offering her roles if she can't do them?" and I said, "Because soon she will be strong enough to do it and I want her to know that I want to work with *her*, not her leg. I want her brain and her talent and I will keep offering her any role at any time to get that."

Plan

Finally, she was ready to go and what a great role to finally have her play. She played Lady Anne in our *Richard III* in 2015 and was marvelous in it, her wonderful talent 'light' undimmed, but now tempered with a new fierceness and a passion and an inner strength that she hadn't maybe fully embraced before her accident. She had also found a strong and vital voice as a writer, speaker and advocate and this strong female role fit the bill for who she was now and who she was becoming.

So, in our cast I opted to include all the actors in the big battle scene, why not? I'm a firm believer that women would fight too! Everyone regardless of age or ability was in the big battle sequence. (This is true of any of our shows that have had a battle sequence over the years, all the artists get to play!)

In thinking about this extended battle I had a momentary vision of Rachel in the midst of battle removing her prosthetic leg and then beating a young man (a lovely Norwegian actor who was a little person named Espen Sigurdsen) to death with it. However, I was also sensitive to not be pushing her into physicality that was new and private to her. So, what did I do? Did I ask her to do it and if so, how? Or did I opt to let it go and not intrude on her as a person by asking her to do something new onstage as an artist? What would you do and how would you do it?

See Chapter 16 for further details of this case study.

7

BLOCKING AND FIGHT SEQUENCES

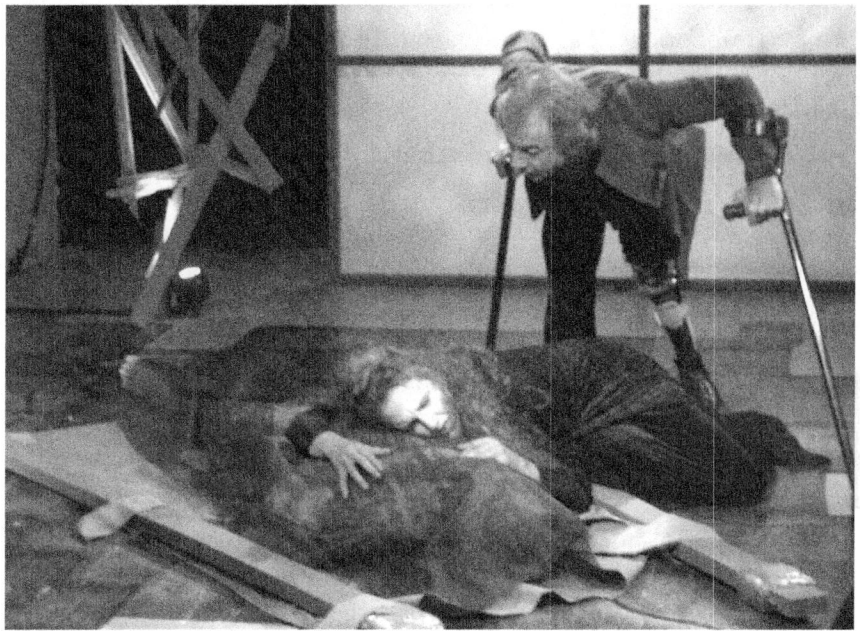

Figure 7.1 Richard III by William Shakespeare, 2007. Henry Holden as Richard and Amber Allison as Lady Anne. (Photograph courtesy of Nicu's Spoon Theater Company.)

In working with artists with disabilities blocking a show is the most immediate and obvious way to break the mold of what the societal and audience normative is. A thorough understanding of how society views disabilities then and what the current norm is has to be where you start. Even playing with the notion of an actor in a wheelchair can deviate from the norms expected if you know what you are starting from and what impact you want to have on the audience. For example, the previously mentioned story about actress Katie Labahn in *How the Day Runs Down* (see Chapter 6). From the opening moment of a dead woman in a wheelchair onstage as the audience filed in, through her re-animating as house lights adjusted, to her dragging herself from the chair and through the audience and out into the lobby, it defied the norms that a wheelchair user must always be in their chair and that it was allowed for the audience to express real horror at her (as she was pretty scary) instead of pity. We then destroy the 'wheelchair etiquette' and the 'pity for the disabled girl' etiquette by doing this.

There are also times where you must adhere to etiquette. Deaf etiquette requires that as you plan out blocking and in any situation where you work with a deaf artist and an interpreter, address the deaf person directly, never the interpreter. The interpreter is a conduit to channel information through, but you always address the deaf artist. The interpreter will not be offended at all. In fact, if you do address the interpreter and not the deaf person it is extremely rude.

Simply stated, the only issue with blocking a blind actor is that she or he cannot see. Simple. That's all. He or she can hear and walk and talk and count paces for blocking and enter arm in arm if coming down stairs or avoiding set pieces. He or she can enter slowly or can be brought on with someone, as opposed to being led. He or she can fight, dance, love, argue and act. There have even been studies on the neuroplasticity of the brain of the visually impaired which show that the blind can utilize echolocation, and that sounds are processed by their visual brain regions as opposed to the auditory regions of the brain. Just get them on the stage and let them do their job. That is *your* job, whether you are a director or an academic recruiter or a casting person.

Using and thinking through ways like this to block plays will lend themselves to the production while still educating the audience away from their preconceived notions. That is why blocking is the very first thing I do after the first read-through as I've said. I liken it to providing a picture frame, both physically and emotionally, so that we can all then paint the entire picture together. It gets all the artists active and then impacts the activity-dependent plasticity of the brain. Blocking can be done in a variety of ways, including counting off steps for artists who are blind and even blocking by color, as in working with an actor on the autism spectrum we put small colored dots on set pieces and blocked him going from color to color because color sequences were what he retained the best. Even if by the performance's opening night the blocking has changed entirely, I always start with grounding the actors into the space and where they move and when. When there are issues of bodies and movement (and even with our non-disabled artists who have memorization problems) it just makes it easier if everyone has a rough idea early on of where they enter, exit and stand onstage.

Speaking of standing, you should always be aware of who can, who cannot and who might not want to. Plays can go on a bit sometimes and you must be aware that Billy has been standing for thirty minutes and oops, should we let him sit? Have chairs where you need them even if it does not go with the 'classic' concept of whatever show you do. Throw the classics out the window if you need to. Add tree stumps, feed bags or boxes as chairs, have your cast explore how to rest onstage or sit onstage and envision what new movement, blocking and body postures you must do so that their bodies can be at home in the world of the play.

If you know you may be forgetting who needs to sit and when, have your stage manager back you up by noting it in the script and reminding you. Also, start at the very beginning of staging to set up and create, or rig if need be, all of your offstage cues for actors, vibrations and sightlines for your deaf artists and any audible or vibratory cues for blind artists, set up prop tables so all actors have access and knives are not at a little person's eye height. Block your show, both on- and offstage, with this in mind always know that something as simple as sending a text from the stage manager to the deaf actor can act as a cue!

For artists with disabilities who often do not get to work, let alone move around onstage, rehearsals should be a physically freeing time. Just because a body is disabled does not mean it cannot move, and move well. Just as artists are always artists, bodies are always bodies, albeit different ones. I have never had a disabled artist who was not able to discover something new physically by just being allowed to move and grow and play. They just need that play room and the safety net of your belief to discover how to move.

Allow for time before the rehearsals for the actors to warm up either in groups or individually. I do not often mandate group warm ups, but sometimes that happens if we are doing a co-played project or if we work with developmentally or mentally disabled artists who need to get some physical energy out. Actors also often pair up, work in small groups or they work alone, but they are given the freedom to find out what warms them up and what works for them. If they need a warm up but do not know how or what to do, we then work with them to give them options or do a group warm up.

Always make sure you have a wide area both onstage and offstage for warm ups and for a wheelchair user (or users, as you may have many wheelchairs in one show) and that they have the room to turn around and be comfortable. Also remove any and all clutter from aisles, floors, walkways, dressing rooms, lobby, box office, any bar or outside intermission area and bathrooms. Often directors may worry about the actor in a wheelchair onstage, but forget that the wheelchair user has to be able to move backstage and turn around, roll down the hall, get in and out of the dressing room, go to the bathroom and wait to enter onstage without blocking other actors, etc. You must know where they can get to easily backstage and onstage before you block them too.

I often get asked if you should say, "OK, now cross down there stage left and saunter over to him" to someone in a wheelchair. You betcha. I've seen actors saunter, sneak, gallop, run, spin, skip and all from their wheelchairs, with canes, crutches or hopping. Their wheelchairs and anything else are a part of them and *are* how they move. Just say the words, ask for what you'd like and let them do the work. It is like the old theatre adage, "Hire good actors and then get out of their way."

When you are creating fight sequences do not shy away from these at all, but do have a certified fight director conduct any fight choreography (if you have union performers, you must have a certified fight director anyway and your insurance requires it as well). Make sure the fight director knows from the beginning who they are working with as that will help him or her to map out the fights in their head. A fight director should be inspired and excited to work with different disabilities as this only opens up a highly creative workspace for everyone. If the fight director is not excited or on board with the process or your artists, then find a new one fast.

Ask at all times of your artists in fight scenes not what they can do, but what are they physically comfortable doing? These may be two very different things. *Then* ask them what they are not comfortable doing. Then ask them if they could do anything else what would it be in the fight scene. Tell them your ideas, offer that first and then see what their response is. Sometimes they will counter your wacky idea with an even wackier one and then you all just figure out how to do it safely. Safety is the main thing, even though you are exploring physicalities.

I am lucky in that I am also a fight director, so in our first production of *Richard III* (in 2007) there is a final battle between Richard and Richmond, ending in Richard's death. We staged the final battle as a pretty epic one as Henry (playing Richard) who had had polio as a child, could be thought of as frail. Hah! In our battle Henry went from arm crutches fighting, to using the crutches as a weapon, to a crutch and a sword (hidden in his crutch), to a dagger,and then finally to hand-to-hand combat and ended up being strangled to death, not stabbed. Our 2015 production of *Richard III* was nearly opposite to this in that the general battle was the epic one, however the final fight between Richard and Richmond happened quickly as Richard III was not at home in his non-disabled body and Richmond was, thus defeating Richard quickly.

Be aware – just in general during the blocking of fight rehearsals – is someone on their feet too long? Do they need time to transition in and out of a wheelchair? Do they need time to gain balance or breathe? If so, build it into the fight. If they can only lie down and fight, then figure that out. How can they fight lying on their back? Do not let small things stop you, keep your mind and theirs working around the issues and finding the way in.

It is also crucial to be aware of medications, food or drink needs and keeping hydrated during fight rehearsals. This is similar to anyone keeping track of things for kids in a kids' show. These actors are not kids, but you may have a list of different needs depending upon the artist. Know each actor's needs and physical limitations and be very careful. How would the body they have behave in a real fight in real life? Map it out and go with it. Trust yourself and them and keep communication open. Discuss with each actor what they can do comfortably and what they might opt to do in a physical situation and construct the fight from their reality which may not necessarily match the script's needs or even your own as a director. Be willing to change your own vision of the play, the fight, the moment, the reality.

Be aware that what they can do not only encompasses the physical, but also the mental and emotional ability to do it (as well as the mental and emotional ability of the audience to understand it). Any of our artists in our rehearsals have the right to stop any rehearsal at any time, not just during fights, by raising a hand for safety issues or for physical reasons. Their concerns are addressed right there on the spot and solved before we move on. Because of the very nature of a disabled body or mind there must be active collaboration and trust and immediate problem solving together or you cannot proceed.

I once choreographed a fight sequence between a blind actor and a sighted one for an informal workshop. Both actors were armed with good balanced swords and the blind actor *always* knew exactly where his hand and full body were in space (much more than the sighted actor did, truthfully) and he knew where to throw his blade so the sighted actor could hit it. The sighted actor was much more tentative and unsure, wrapped in his pity, not wanting to 'hurt the blind guy,' but the blind actor had it down and was amazing. I had to stop and tell the sighted actor to ramp it up as his 'pity' was getting his butt kicked. I say this to illustrate that the disabled body may not be the one you have the most problems with at all, it may often be the non-disabled ones.

Another little person who has worked with us over the years is Colin Buckingham, an avid swordsman and fight lover, who was in our 2015 production of *Red Noses*. I told him, get certified as a fight director. First, and most importantly, because he is very good at being a fight director. Second because the fight world needs a little person who is an excellent fight choreographer and defies any and all stereotypes. Third, because he understands how many different types of bodies move through space, and that is sadly often a rare thing even in a fight director. I know I would hire him anytime to choreograph fights for me.

Nothing is impossible. That sounds trite, but I do not just say that, I actually know it to be true. It is only that the disabled body uses a different set of reference points in space and time when it works. The disabled mind does the same. Then we may have to extrapolate that every time to each different disability as they each use a different set of references. This is a great part of the wonder of it all for me as I get a chance to follow how each different mind works and what their references are. This teaches all of us new ways to perceive things and then slowly we can begin to get it. To get each other. To get together.

Most artists with disabilities are *keenly* aware of where their bodies are in space and in relationship to others. We have a wonderful actor, Sammy Mena (mentioned in Chapter 4), who has been with our company for years and who always knows where he is in space and what his body is doing although he is legally blind. He has a heightened sense of his relationship to space and air currents and his hearing is also eerily marvelous as he constantly amazes us with his eavesdropping talents. His reference points are air currents at times, and shadows at other times. Even within his own abilities the reference points may often change which is a good thing to remember.

A note about when or if you have a blind artist enter with another artist: do not have them led onstage unless the role calls for it. There is an etiquette about this, where the sighted person offers the crook of their arm or even their forearm and the blind person can then rest their hand where it is comfortable. There can be variations on this, lord knows we have done all kinds of things, but the variations need to be worked out with an eye to being respectful of the artist, but true to the role. Dragging a blind person on is as obnoxious as dragging anyone on, but is also insulting to the blind community.

Another thing to also be aware of is the newness of the disability (were they born with it and know nothing else? Are they newly, within the last three years, disabled?) These are *very* different places to be both mentally and physically and will have a big impact on what their reference points for movement are and how used to their disabled body they are. A newly disabled artist may need you to help them find their body and balance and adjusted capacity for work or stress or movement or stamina, or assistance in assessing their new ways of thinking of and referencing of their body onstage or during various phases of movement. Do not assume that they do need help, though. The assumption that all individuals with disabilities want and constantly need help without actually asking the person if they do is an ableist error. They will tell you if they need help or you can ask, but never assume.

It sounds complicated, but it is very easy. Experiment and encourage, help them physically if you are asked to by standing behind them and holding them and letting them find balance points.

Dance with them. Do what they need. Let them listen and move and do what they need to do physically to find themselves in the world you make even if it doesn't always work. Let the actor try and fail and try and half-fail and then try and succeed. Give them a place of safety so they can create with you.

Case Study 7: Think Outside the Box, Nicu's Spoon Theater, New York City

History

In 2005 we produced a play by Mark Medoff (best known for the Oscar winning *Children of a Lesser God*), the previously mentioned *Stumps* (the play itself had two disabled roles in it) and we created a new performance style I termed co-playing. My idea in 2005 (after gestating for a few years) was that there had to be something beyond interpreting for the deaf (now Deaf West in LA does shadowed work with artists somewhat similar to co-playing) where a pair of artists would play one role, one hearing and one deaf, one signing and one speaking, but *both* acting, owning and interpreting the role simultaneously. I was also wanting to create a performance format where our deaf audiences and our hearing audiences (as we had loads of both) could attend the same performances and watch the play together, laugh together, cry together and be together throughout a performance so that the line between deaf and hearing audiences was blurred and could quite possibly not exist for that brief span of time. Our co-played shows also, from the beginning, had full runs. The co-playing was not just a one- or two-night occasion, but was how the entire show and run of the show was structured, thus deaf audiences could attend at any time.

In the first project we did this we had the deaf artists play the inner persona and the speaking artists play the outer persona. This required a partnership onstage which demands constant communication, physical closeness (as on occasion the blocking may be very physical and almost choreographed) real care and a heightened awareness of your partner. We since have done two other co-played productions where we threw out all our previous notions about our own co-playing and continued to re-envision more new styles and ways for the artists to co-own a role.

We needed various locations for the ten actors in *Stumps* (two in each of the five roles). The original set idea was that the actor(s) in the wheelchair would be on ground level. We began work with that and figuring out the complicated movement patterns for ten actors (mostly getting them from ideas or images inside my head into me verbally communicating them, then it being translated into ASL and then all of us making it a reality onstage) and I worked us into possible options to think outside the box.

Plan

This was a show about combining two types of theatre, theatre for hearing and theatre for deaf audiences at the same time. The movement was very specific as we had the pairing of actors to work with. We had an actor in a wheelchair so that was an added thing to take into account. Plus we also needed constant clean sightlines for the audience for the signing actors to be seen, In addition one pairing of two artists played a veteran in a wheelchair and one pairing played a veteran who had a prosthetic hand. So, what could we do to turn it all more on its head and go against expectations?

See Chapter 16 for further details of this case study.

Chapter Action: A Seven-Point List of How You Would Proceed to do a Cast Dance for a Period Play

You have in your cast two actors who are blind and two others with mobility issues and another artist is a little person and another artist has low-scale autism. Think through at least seven steps you must put in place in order to complete the dance for the stage. These may involve the artists, music, production issues, staging or costuming and choreography and are not comprehensive, only ten things you must do within this process. Answers and many variations on this idea will be up to your imagination.

8

COSTUMES, PROPS AND MAKEUP

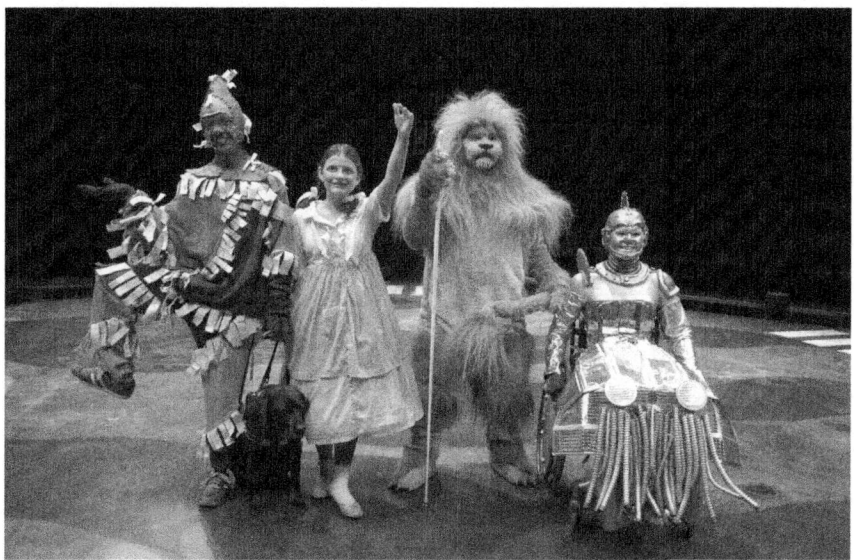

Figure 8.1   *The Wiz* by Charlie Smalls and William F. Brown, 2006. Juliet Villa as
Dorothy, Regan Linton as the Tin Girl, Don Mauck as the Cowardly
Lion, Daniel Traylor as the Scarecrow and Deidra as Toto. (Photograph
courtesy of Phamaly Theatre Company.)

Costumes, props and makeup. Time and again they can be the
key element that can make a character complete. Thus, using the
accessible theory that all things can be made to work for all artists
at all times and to enhance all artists, you can and should adjust
the story, casting, costumes, blocking, makeup, fights, music, cues,
lights, set and stage to the actors' needs. You will note I did not say
alter the text, not unless you have the right to do so.

Oddly, as well as not altering the text, there will be scripts you
will encounter that will prohibit cross-gender casting or color-aware

(which I prefer to the incorrect 'color blind') casting, but you will never run into scripts which prohibit artists who are disabled. You can, indeed, appeal and request cross-gender or color-aware casting, an all female *Glengarry Glen Ross* (by David Mamet) happened after years of David Mamet not granting approval for it. You can make your case to the author or rights holders. Moreover, if you have the playwright present (as with a new script) or get special permission you can even alter the text which can help with outdated terms or other needs.

"Oh it must be so limiting." I often hear from young, new costume or set designers about designing for artists with disabilities. The exact opposite has proven to be true time and time again. When you have a body that does not fit the status quo, or that has additional elements like a wheelchair, crutches, a blind stick, etc., it compels your designers to not think or design for the status quo. How freeing that has been for our designers, to have no limits on their ideas as they design costumes or a set. They can then add in outrageous ideas, adjustable (changeable with different body shapes, types, moments, transitions) clothing, use types of fabrics they might not usually use, use buttons and zippers and lots of velcro that is adaptive to different body needs and kinetics.

In costuming make sure each actor can move in the very specific way their body needs to move in the show and within their specific character comfort zone. Incorporate wheelchairs (and no long sleeves for costumes for manual 'push' wheelchair users, for crying out loud!), crutches and prosthetics into the costumes and props (can they use their arm crutches or a part of their wheelchair as weapons? Can an arm extended with a crutch in it become the large wing of an angel?) and into the makeup for each role. I cannot tell you how transforming it was when we did a play about zombies, *How the Day Runs Down* by John Langan, and Sammy Mena was finally able to do a role without his fake eye. After a life of prosthetics he got a chance to operate freely and act without it if he chose to. Note the word 'chose.' I did not tell him to remove his prosthetic eye as to be a cool zombie (as he was pretty scary already in drag as a female zombie) I gave him the choice as to whether he wanted to work with the fake eye out and he did.

Creative designers can even incorporate additional lighting into the wheelchairs and allow for some traveling or spinning light effects. Wheelchairs, crutches, canes and prosthetics, in fact, can provide some of the best inspirations for new costume, set or lighting ideas. A body part of an artist can become a focal point of a light change or start of an act or scene. You must use your creativity and the artist's creativity and invite and support and challenge your designers to think outside the box. I always invite all designers to attend any and all rehearsals (and depending upon the schedule do have nights when they *must* attend) as I know once they see the rehearsal and development process we have, *really* see it and understand it, they immediately say, "Oh my gosh, where is my pen? I need to write this idea down!" and thus they start having new ideas like mad. This also trains and reinforces a young designer's brain to be continually open to new creative thoughts and new artists and bodies. Many of these designers go on to work at large regional theatres or commercial venues and I want them to be vocal advocates (whether they themselves are disabled or not) for inclusion anywhere they work in the future. Their becoming advocates can only happen if they learn it working with my company or other companies who do this work.

With inclusive companies we never costume to hide disabilities, races, ages, colors or anything else unless it is a plot point we want to either emphasize or to reveal to the audience later. Costumes most of the time should enhance your players and their work, the players are cast for their talent and uniqueness so their costumes are not meant to cover up that uniqueness. Remind your artists that their bodies are beautiful by how you dress them, when appropriate. Adhere to their comfort levels. Twice in my directing life I have had an artist who was disabled request that I take their costume measurements as they did not have a high enough level of comfort with the costume designer. One of those times I honored that request (there were personal reasons for it which had nothing to do with the designer and everything to do with the artist) and the other time we talked through the request with the designer and the artist's nerves dissipated and all was fine. Adhere to their comfort levels.

Also take note if you need to have dressers backstage for various artists during the show. Plan this from the beginning so you know how many bodies are where and when. We usually will have, with a large cast show, one rehearsal about two weeks from opening where the stage manager *only* focuses on tracking all the costume changes. Where are costume changes and when and who does them and do they need help? Both offstage and on all actors must feel supported and as low-stress as possible. Keep in mind that what stresses one artist may not stress another. Various autistic actors may need to have softer or less noisy fabrics for costumes, while non-autistic artists may not, so be aware of this and make sure the designers are too. Assure your cast of the laundry days during your show as well so they do not stress, or have any worry or body odor issues about that. For any obsessive-compulsive disorder (OCD) or autism spectrum disorders (ASD) involving body odors, or perceived body odors, have them use underarm pads which are removable and disposable each night and also prolong the life of the costume.

Any prosthetic limbs should also either be covered by pants, dress or whatever (as opposed to being wrapped in something which will tangle), or if left exposed, should be able to operate freely (we costumed a young woman with a prosthetic leg in a long dress and just pinned her dress up in front, steampunk style, so that her leg was fully free to move). There is nothing worse than having a prosthetic limb caught in something costumed onstage (except maybe a costume stuck in a wheelchair wheel or electric wheelchair mechanism). Artists who are sight impaired actually are easily the most adept at finding things offstage and changing (even with numerous quick prop or costume changes) without help, all by feel, and usually anyone attempting to assist them just gets in their way and costs them time so do not make assumptions based on your idea of the disability. When in doubt, ask.

The technical aspects (costume, sets, lights, props, makeup, sound and music, multimedia elements) need to support the artists. So must you and your staff. Personal props for artists can also be incorporated into certain prosthetics or wheelchairs. I was once choreographing a fight scene for *Richard III*, in 2015, where I had an artist (the late and much missed Joe Genera) in a 'push' wheelchair chase a non-disabled actor (Perri Yaniv) onstage at full blast and I was pondering what he could kill Perri with, but I didn't know quite where to mount a sword or dagger on his wheelchair. Joe looked at me and said, "Well, I could kill him with this" and pulled off a broken part of his wheelchair back, a long, metal scary thing. We shined it up a bit and oiled it to be sure it came off smoothly (and really couldn't kill Perri) and we had a murder weapon.

In our first production of *Richard III* in 2007 (which I did not direct, but did produce) we had an extra arm crutch (we had three arm crutch sets for Richard in this play) used only in the final fight between Richard and Richmond because we had hollowed it out and put a removable sword in it for Richard III to whip out. It was a very cool moment, and it brought audible gasps from the audience every night. Use what you and they have to work with and let the artist tell you their ideas. I had had the idea for the sword in the crutch effect but didn't have the extra crutches and it was not until dear Henry (playing Richard) said "Oh god, I must have five or six pairs of old arm crutches if we need them!" that I realized we could possibly make it work.

So, what if you have a company that only does children's theatre? How then do you cast disabled artists without alienating audiences, children and parents? Do you have fears you will bother or scare the children? Do you worry you will make parents uncomfortable? We have done six children's shows out of our forty mainstage plays and we have *never* had issues of that nature. We have actually had great responses like this:

> What I liked was Nicu's Spoon Theater's wonderfully straightforward version of inclusion. Actress and playwright Katie Labahn performs in a wheelchair—it's not a plot point, nor is the character described that way; there is simply no reason why Lady Malcolm (or any other character in the play really) shouldn't be in a wheelchair. When she entered, my daughter turned to me and asked if the actress really needed a wheelchair? I nodded, she nodded and turned back to watch the show. That moment was a far more valuable lesson than when the performers turned to the kids in the audience and told them that lying is bad and gets you into trouble.
>
> Rohana Elias-Reyes, nytheatre.com

Or this:

> Your productions are so well geared to my student body from our 1st graders to our 5th graders, they all love them. Your integrated use of actors with disabilities has also made your productions

great for my Special Education Students as well as my General Ed Students as they see themselves reflected onstage.

Laurie Greenwald, Theater Teacher, PS 50

So, stop worrying and get to doing and creating and writing and casting. Children are the best audiences you will ever have because they truly believe a paper puppet is really a butterfly and they just do not worry about a disability unless we teach them to. The more they see it isn't an issue the more their perception of the world and of other different beings grows. If the children in the audience have disabilities as well then it is pure joy, sometimes so intense that it brings them to tears, when they see themselves reflected onstage. It is vital that our young disabled artists have solid, talented and supported role models so these kids can have the solid belief that they too can be artists. For non-disabled children as well it is a good educational experience to encounter talented and vibrant artists with disabilities just like they will encounter in the real world.

Case Study 8: Opening the Door, Phamaly Theatre, Denver, Colorado

Design concepts at Phamaly Theatre Company, Case by Bryce Alexander, Artistic Director through mid 2016

History

Phamaly Theatre Company (formerly known as The Physically Handicapped Actors & Musical Artists League) produces professional-scale plays and musicals year-round throughout the Denver, Colorado Metro region, cast entirely of performers with disabilities across the spectrum (physical, cognitive, emotional, blindness, deafness, etc.). Phamaly was formed in 1989 when five students of the Boettcher School in Denver, Colorado, grew frustrated with the lack of theatrical opportunities for people living with disabilities, and decided to create a theatre company that would provide individuals with disabilities the opportunity to perform onstage.

One of the largest hesitations for the use of an actor with a disability in traditional theatre is the fear of the physical limitations an actor might bring to the design process. How can you build a scenic element with multiple steps if an actor is in a wheelchair, for example? The reality, however, is that the astounding set of possibilities that an actor with a disability provides often results in higher quality, more creative, and highly effective design elements. Over the last twenty-eight seasons, Phamaly Theatre Company has seen a number of high-profile design and staging concepts that have illustrated the value of artistic inclusion.

Perhaps the most striking example of effective use of disability theory in the design process came during Phamaly's 2006 production of *The Wiz*. Cast in the leading roles were a Dorothy who was blind; a Scarecrow who was hearing impaired; a Lion who was blind; and a Tin-girl in a wheelchair. At first glance, this set of actors seemed to defy the standard expectation of the 'embodiment' of each character.

Plan

Inspired by the qualities of each performer, costume designer Mallory Nelson had as her task to design and incorporate profound costume elements that would not only serve the actors, but the play, as well.

While the results discussed in the outcomes are just two examples of the many design features and accessibility concepts built into this particular production, the lesson is clear: Small inclusion can make a big impact. When these design elements were combined with Dorothy's guide dog as Toto, and a tap-dance included through tin-cans on the hands of the Tin-girl, the production was highly memorable and the production value exceptional. As the *Denver Post* theatre critic John Moore wrote at the time:

> What's most moving may be inadvertent. Of course it's not written for Dorothy to ask the Wiz to see, or for the Tin Girl to walk, so they don't. But this omission tells the story of Phamaly far better than *The Wiz* ever could – they all believe in themselves, just the way they are.

Other examples of clear and specific use of concept include an executive chorus of entirely blind actors in *Urinetown*, all of whom had matching glasses; an intentionally wheelchair inaccessible platform in the center of the unit-set for *Glass Menagerie*; and a scenic design and director's concept for *Joseph and the Amazing Technicolor Dreamcoat* that implied the cast were trapped in an institution and working together to remember that 'any dream will do.'

See Chapter 16 for further details of this case study.

9

TECHNICAL REHEARSALS AND
FINAL DRESS

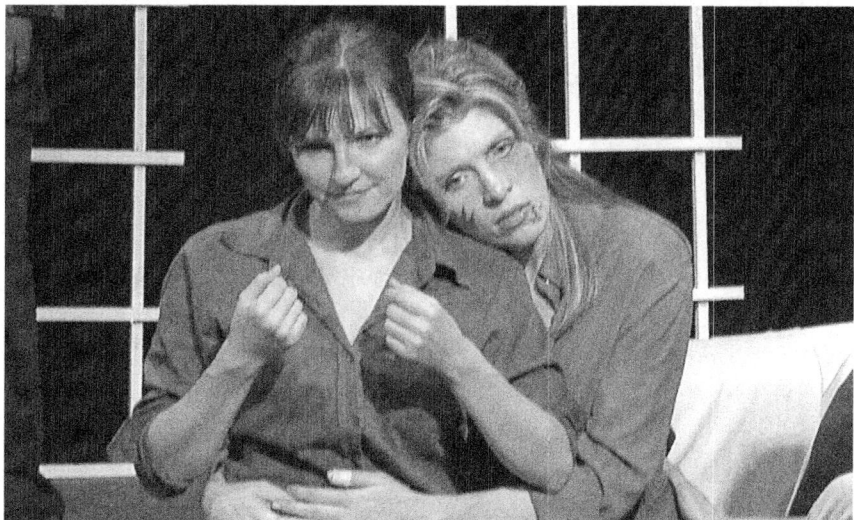

Figure 9.1   *Stumps* by Mark Medoff, 2005. L to R Kate Breen and Thea McCartan.
(Photograph courtesy of Nicu's Spoon Theater Company.)

Director Stephanie Barton-Farcas, also artistic director of Nicu's
Spoon Theater Company, told Playbill.com that the production
is designed to ask, "What is disability?" She said, "Our mission
is to create dialogue and re-envision plays people think they
know." In doing the production, Barton-Farcas puts her troupe
squarely in the middle of the current debate about whether
disabled characters should ever be played by non-disabled actors.
She added, "Some of the actors are very forthcoming about
themselves while others are deeply private and we go by what
their comfort level is. One of our youngest actors Estelle Olivia

has a persistent spine condition which at times puts her in intense pain, but to all who see her she would seem non-disabled."

Robert Viagas, *Playbill*, 2015

The day of loading in or set build in a theatre, your technical rehearsal and final dress rehearsal is the most difficult, crazed and stressful time of any production. Once you and your crew load into the theatre or get that set built and ready, and as you enter your technical rehearsal, always leave your mind open to new ideas even as you are busy building the set and running technical cues at the last moment. Consider using your artists within the show to incorporate lights beyond the onstage practicals (like using hand-held flashlights, LED finger lights, actor controlled and operated light sources, headlamps, Christmas tree lights, emergency lighting aspects, light-up shoes or props, glow in the dark costumes, makeup or puppets, etc.)

Most importantly as you work and tweak and finalize cues and so forth be very time aware – are the artists standing or sitting too long? Your cast is aware (and if not, if they are newer to theatre, then prepare them by letting them know tech night will be five or more hours long) of how long the night will be, but plan accordingly. I always call actors to arrive at the theatre after the stage is set and sound levels are set and make additional provisions for actors who need to arrive early to just have some private time on the new set walking, entering, exiting and being in the space. Be aware of their stress levels, which for some may be at a higher level than for a non-disabled artist. Be aware of who is returning to the stage after a long absence or who is making a debut. We add in extra time for all actors as well for the fight sequences and dances before the general cast call to the theatre. This extra time and checking in is built into our load-in day and our technical schedule for the artists who need it.

Your company should make it a standard company or theatre policy to have accessible sets (wide entrances and exits, ramps, all cleared of any obstacles) and remember all sets with wheelchairs on the stage must have turnaround points *both* on- and offstage and/ or near ramps. Having sets and onstage set pieces (tables, chairs) with very defined corners as well is very helpful to your blind artists. They need defined places to ground themselves and set as reference points. If you intend on doing performances for audience members who are blind you will need your set to be accessible to them for the pre-show tactile tours as well. If a set element is not well defined and accessible then there should be an artistic, staging or project vision (or even budgetary) reason. You can make a point onstage just as well by having areas or set pieces that are not accessible to an actor or actors, just be sure it is by artistic choice, not by neglect.

Be sure to run complicated sound and light cues with the stage manager and ASMs and yourself as stand-ins and set all your sound cues at some rough levels approximately where you think they should be so that by the time you do add the actors you only need to double-check and tweak the sound and light cues. Of course, nothing is ever perfect, especially during the technical rehearsals, but you can minimize the wear and tear and stress on your actors by putting the bulk of the technical work on yourself, your staff, volunteers and crew. Production assistants or volunteers and interns are always on call for load-in and early technical runs as they can stand in for actors as lights are focused and they can help you to set sound cues as you can listen to the cues with real bodies on the stage. Your disabled artists will know that tech night will be hard on them, but if you have picked the right tech staff and designers and actors and thoroughly prepared them, they will all be more than up to the task.

Be heavily aware of physical needs during technical nights. Keep water and snacks available or ask the actors to bring them. We work with all ages in our shows so we try to be aware of our older artists as well as our young kids in the cast. I always feed actors (pizza!!) at the technical rehearsals as well as at the first read. Because we work with many diverse artists we often end up with a potluck of different foods which they bring on our tech night too. Never underestimate the inherent power of sitting and breaking bread together. Never underestimate the time to eat and talk and share.

You should have had props and any weaponry *way* before your final tech rehearsal (as a policy we add props and weapons and fight work or dance pretty soon after we rough stage everything – say by week two of rehearsals at the latest) and your actors should have had their costumes settled and had final fittings done at least a week before final tech as well. Never add a weapon or important prop at the last moment if you can help it, that is asking for trouble. This is a hard and fast rule that applies with or without artists with disabilities in the cast.

How and when to set up your production and cast photos depends upon you and your marketing needs and deadlines, but I would recommend doing it as soon as you have costumes even remotely wearable (and sometimes even without costumes or a set if you have to) so that they can be used in press packets and advertising and in any articles or interviews. Also keep in mind that nowadays social media, streaming sites like YouTube or personal websites and the internet in general rules everything, so the sooner your cast and public relations (PR) staff can have approved digital photos the sooner they will be all over the internet and in the news. Once you are in tech however, I recommend more photos or shots of any moments you have missed or that are particularly stunning.

An important thing to remember if you work in inclusion or disability theatre, or at least something that we have been careful about, is not cropping or allowing to be cropped photos of your cast and their bodies. Our company does not allow the cropping or photoshopping out of crutches, wheelchairs, etc. (Although if truth be told we have only had to strongly ask for this once in our history.) Full body shots stay full body shots, and all you have to do is mention this to the interviewer or make a note in the press packet that you must be asked before cropping of photos is done. The gorgeous bodies and faces of your artists are not to be hidden or shown in half light, wheelchairs or crutches or stumps or canes or scars are not to be cropped out, they are to be included. Inclusion is the point.

Make the time in your photo shoot to get comprehensive group shots and at least one solid shot of each artist in action. If you have never planned a photoshoot before, there is a template on the companion website. This photo shoot goes beyond your company PR needs and goes to the artists' and designers' own memories, websites, portfolios and their future career and work. If your staff or designers are artists with disabilities (and even if they are not) be sure to get many full stage shots or great lighting moments or costume shots for their portfolios. The entire process is meant to grow all of them as working professional artists and enable them to have solid tools to be competitive in future jobs. So, make the time to do a thorough photo shoot so that they have great pictures of the performance to show for all their hard work. You can even ask them if there are particular moments that they feel are special or pivotal to their work and plan those shots into your photo call list.

Case Study 9: A Large Disabled and Diverse Cast in Technical Rehearsal, Nicu's Spoon Theater, New York City

History

We entered technical rehearsal for our 2015 production of *Red Noses* which I had adored (when the endless logistics and giant cast size didn't drive me wacky) directing. Our largest cast ever – twenty-six – was one of our most diverse as well. With a fifty-year age span and various colors and disabilities, a wonderful text, and eight live musical numbers, it was a dream fulfilled for a director who dreams big like me. The set was a motley collection of graffiti with a post-apocalyptic feel (as we had translated the black plague into modern day New York City) and the Monty Python-ish black comedy feel of the work allowed us much leeway in playing through how the cast's disabilities impacted the play and the roles.

For instance, at one point a possible battle was to ensue between four motley fellows, one of whom was a little person, Colin Buckingham. All four drew swords and faced off and the actor opposite Colin did a double-take and then dropped to his knees to match Colin's stature. Or when we played with audio perception and had a phone ring mid-show (in the play within a play section of the text) which sent actors into the audience, swords drawn, and then sheepishly back to the stage when it was revealed to be a cast member.

In the closing sequence of the play we had plans to use a fog machine. We had not used it in rehearsal (although we had talked it through with the cast) and it was only going to be used for a very short sequence at the end of the show. We knew we would have to run it during tech with the full cast in order to even see if it would work well with that many bodies onstage. However, our youngest actor was five and our oldest in their seventies and we had varying breathing and bronchial and medical issues in the cast. How could we use the fog machine in tech rehearsal? This is very different from during performance. In performance it runs for fifteen seconds, the sequence happens and the play ends and we open the doors immediately to air it out. In technical rehearsal we could possibly run it for an hour or more.

Plan

During our technical rehearsal however, we needed to test it in many ways. How long should it run? How much fog came from where and went where? Where should the fog machine even be situated? How thick was the fog? How fast could we make it dissipate? What would it even look like? There was much testing to be done. So, how did we do it? Without mangling the cast we hope, but still being able to get the information we needed to use it each night, again without hospitalizing any member of the cast?

See Chapter 16 for further details of this case study.

10

PUBLIC RELATIONS AND MARKETING

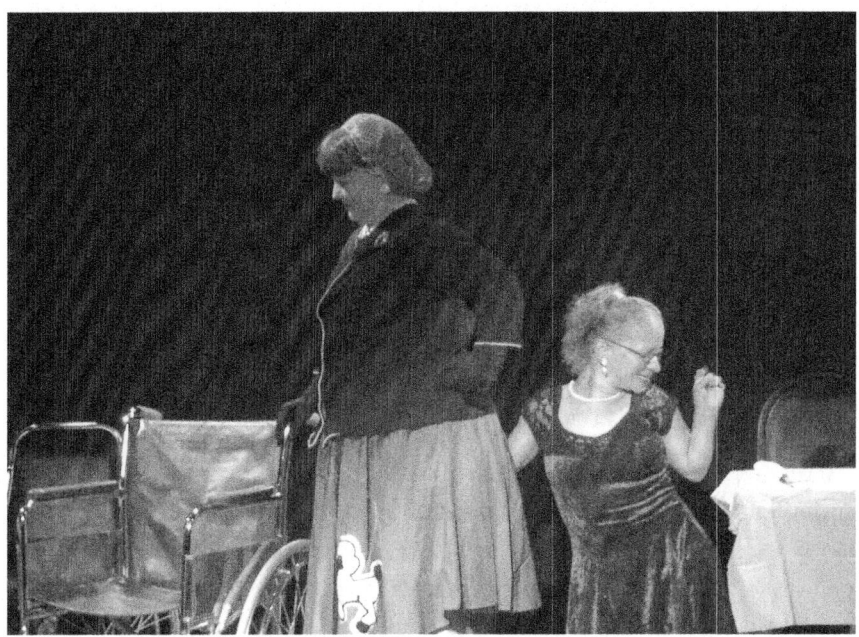

Figure 10.1 Kosher Harry by Nick Grosso, 2007. L to R Wynne Anders and Shira Grabelsky co- playing 'The Old Woman.' (Photograph courtesy of Nicu's Spoon Theater Company.)

The work they (Nicu's Spoon) are doing is passionate, professional and absolutely worth keeping an eye on.

Theatre Scene, 2003, Tim Browning

A fast and important note about online and digital public relations. If you do not know how to upload, manage and link or embed your YouTube videos and your pictures and reviews to your company's own website, Facebook page (you have a Facebook page for your company and event, right?) and social media pages, or if you do not have a website at all, then you *must* create one. You must have a 'digital footprint' for your company and for each single production. Anyone who offers to volunteer for you who has webpage experience can create and maintain your website or teach one of your permanent staff how to do it. Have your webmaster and staff read technical assistance documents like 'Accessibility of State and Local Government Websites to People with Disabilities' (listed in the resources) to help them out on how to plan it. Have links to ticketing, reviews and resources if needed, but do have a website.

Make certain that your website can be as accessible as your performance and rehearsal spaces (and this is difficult as new technologies are coming faster than you will be able to get them online). Production photos, production history, reviews, your mission statement, press announcements, audition notices; all of this and more must be front and center online for funders, audience, actors and artists to see and hear. This is a digital age in every way and your company must not only be online but must be keeping up.

Rule number two of PR and marketing for an inclusive company or show is to be aware of and keep serious control over (as much as you can) the tone of writing about your disabled cast and staff. Include information in your interviews and press releases that educate, like: "A recent study by the Ruderman Family Foundation found that ninety-five percent of roles that depict characters with disabilities on television are played by able-bodied actors, while a University of Southern California study reports that of the top hundred films, forty-five films included no characters with disabilities. This, despite the fact that disabled people make up twenty percent of the population." Dropping these issues and tidbits into your interviews shows the investment you make in this work. If this work becomes important to your group then you must educate and know what you are discussing with the press.

You control what you put out to a great extent, but also you will have to teach and be very up front with the press or interviewers about the fact that these are seasoned actors and should be addressed as such. There are no 'pity articles' about my company, nor any "Golly aren't we all great and brave and inspiring! Give us a hand!" articles because that is not what we put out or stand for. You may even, as we have at times, discuss with interviewers or reviewers the correct language and terms they should use or the types of disabilities they will be seeing on the stage. As much as you can, be in control of how your artists, show and company are perceived. This is not a theatre of feeling sorry for folks, not a theatre of let's applaud because we feel bad for them, this is professional theatre with artists who should be as respected as any other company would be. The respect, by the way, starts with you and how you approach the press and reviewers and ultimately, the audience, about your work. They all take their cues from you, remember that.

In 2016 one of my favorite disabled activists, scholars, speaker/ teachers and handsome men about town, Lawrence Carter-Long, conducted a workshop on doing better disability stories for and with professional journalists at the 2016 Excellence in Journalism conference in New Orleans. This was on behalf of the National Council on Disability (where Lawrence works) and along with Lawrence were, in his words, "the most excellent tag-team partners Lily Altavena and David Perry." Training like this is vital for the journalists, but you as an educator or theatre practitioner must take matters upon yourself and educate when needed. Lawrence Carter-Long is one of the best resources in the US for this type of training and seminar.

Often you must also address accessibility issues in your public relations, interviews, press packets, company website and ticket sales websites or even telephone messages. The onus is on you to ensure that audiences understand how to get tickets, where and when to arrive for certain types of access (wheelchair users may enter at a different door than those on foot, for instance, or may be able to take a regular or freight elevator) and how to let you know at any time what their needs are. When we are in production my cell phone is an active conduit to any disabled audience member who needs anything.

Also be aware of which actors/staff or designers are comfortable talking about their life as a disabled artist in a PR situation or in interviews. If you do not have a good idea about this then just ask them. Some artists want to just be actors or designers and not discuss their disabilities in an open forum for the press, and other artists welcome the chance to discuss their life as an artist with a disability and you should know which ones are which. There are even artists with disabilities who choose not to identify as an artist with a disability, just only as an artist. I do not judge any of their choices in how they view themselves at all and it always their choice, but you can be certain I know who is who within my cast and staff so I do not recommend an interviewer talk to the wrong artist. However it works out, you or your PR person need to know and then deal with any interview requests accordingly.

Examples of your own company history that can and should be included in a press kit (these are given out to press, reviewers and interviewers) can be reviews of past productions, complete with photographs, past interviews with you and/or company members or other actors, any spotlight or local community television or video pieces on your company. (You can even put any television or video clips on a CD and include video and audio clips in your press packet.) You can add a CD with high resolution quality photos from your recent photo shoot of the current show (thus they can put them right into their articles and not have to contact you further for photographs). This again also enables easier control of your photos not being cropped. If your company has been honored with any past awards, whether for their work and investment in the neighboring community or for their artistic work, you can include articles reflecting this or even a list of the awards and when and why they were given.

One last, and seemingly odd, thought about PR and marketing: do not discount the power of friends and families of any of your performers and designers. Those artists with disabilities who have the love and support of their families (many do not, unfortunately) usually have a machine of activity and support behind them. We have had families take flyers and postcards and cover the city, get group bookings for us, call and make contacts interview or review us. Do not discount the support that is around you and your cast and staff. If families want to help, let them! For a family to see their loved one return to the arts after a disabling incident, or see their child with a disability (who may not have been given opportunities in school or otherwise) enter the arts and blossom is an overwhelming experience and one they deserve to be an active part of if they wish. When support and help are offered, take it and say a gracious 'thank you'.

Case Study 10: Phamaly Theatre Company, Denver, Colorado

Bryce Alexander, Artistic Director for Case Study; Regan Linton, Artistic Director as of late 2016

History

In *Man of La Mancha,* the character of Aldonza is taken from her horse, savagely raped and beaten, and left to die. In many high-budget productions, the actress has been taken from a live horse onstage. Phamaly's 2009 production of *Man of La Mancha* could not feature a live horse. But Regan Linton, a wheelchair user and the actress playing Aldonza, was able to more effectively portray her character's struggle and abuse with more impact than any other production the audience had seen.

Plan

Audiences at Phamaly often comment on their quick acceptance of an actor's disability within their character, and within the world of the play.

When Aldonza lost the freedom provided by her wheelchair, the audience concretely understood what had truly been taken from her in the previous scene. But Regan's willingness made the production one of the most highly regarded and recounted in our twenty-eight-year history.

See Chapter 16 for further details of this case study.

Chapter Action: Create your PR and Marketing Plan

(This is provided in depth on the website in separate checklists.)

What items might you include in a press kit? Which artists and designers in your cast are available for interviews? Which of the pictures show off the cast and show as a whole and how can you tell the good pictures from the bad? What statement do you want to make about your work and company as part of your press kit? What kinds of audiences, nationalities or special communities do you want to contact? (Maybe you have a Brazilian artist in your show. If so, you would be silly to not invite the Brazilian community and to talk about that in the press. Also invite disabled groups and organizations, support groups, learning centers and community groups.) Who are all the special guest artists you want to talk about? What can you say that will enable artists and staff to use this event to move on to more work? How can you enhance their work and reputation? What do you want the play to say as a whole about you and your theatre? What past articles, interviews, reviews, brochures, newsletters or information can also be included in your press packet? What can be in your press kit that can work for the future as opposed to for just this show? (For example, links to your website and mailing list sign ups, asking for donations, volunteers, a wish list of items or needs for the season, etc.)

Be sure to remember to include the normal things in this press kit that you would give to your audiences like a program for the current show and any other materials or inserts for that program.

11

THE PERFORMANCE RUN AND STRIKE

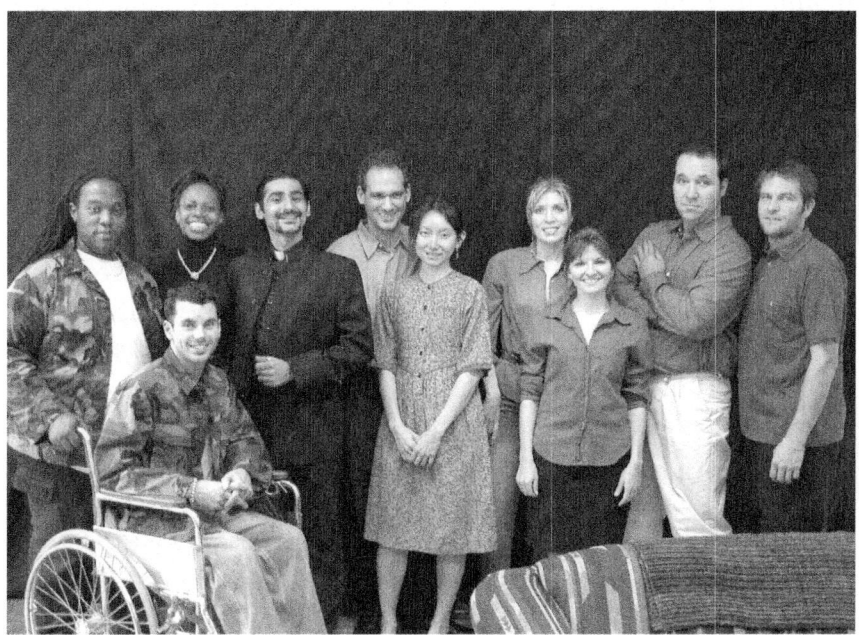

Figure 11.1 *Stumps* by Mark Medoff, 2005. L to R Tyson Jennette, Alvaro Sena in wheelchair, Pamela O. Mitchell, Karam Puri, Paul Savas, Jovinna Chan, Thea McCartan, Kate Breen, T.J. Mannix and Darren Frazier. (Photograph courtesy of Nicu's Spoon Theater Company.)

Everyone, if they live long enough, will become disabled. It is the one minority class which anyone can become a member of at anytime.

> Playwright John Belluso, *The San Francisco Observer*, 2005 interview

To what extent are performers with disabilities able to challenge and thus subvert the ingrained 'rules' of theatrical and film society? What would a stage performance look like without a societal ideology of theatrical ability? What about with no ideology about disability in theatre or film at all? How then does a disabled artist speaking a line give it more resonance or a new and different resonance than an able-bodied actor? How can a disabled body illuminate a text, a role or a physical movement in a new way? These and other creative and socially challenging questions are only a few that a performance run can fully awaken and explore.

Once you have opened your show you can finally settle down and relax into a good run. My company usually does a three-week run minimum (which is long for New York City as many of the theatres do one week or even as little as three to four shows after a full month of rehearsal, unless of course, you are on Broadway), however many regional theatres may run a month, six weeks or longer, so that the artists can grow into their roles, the designers and crew can get a good run and so that the reviewers and local awards judges will come. Be very aware of the best reviewers in your city and how long a performance run you need in order to guarantee their attendance. In New York City, and in most large cities, you need to run over two weeks if you want the larger reviewers to attend like *The New York Times* and *Playbill*.

During your run of performances and your end-of-show strike keep on top of all the things that have been discussed plus adding in any new visual, vibratory and text cues during the run (always be ready to tweak any cues), and use of telephones, sight, lights and shadows to cue. If you have any added performances during your run with ASL interpreting, as we usually do, be sure to have a co-box office person out in front who is fluent in ASL. We are lucky in that we have a company member, Bram Weiser, who is extraordinary at this and a charmer to all audiences. We also always reserve a large block of seats with the best visual sightlines for the deaf patrons on those dates and add a general extra wash of lights to the stage lighting for those performances to ensure good visuals for the audience to see the interpreters. An additional tip is to never have blackouts in the normal places for an ASL show, but to hold any light cues specifically for the ASL interpreters during the performance. They cannot interpret in the blackout and I cannot count the times I have seen an ASL show where there were no terp lights (we have even added clip lights for ASL performances if needed in a pinch) and no eliminating or cutting to half light of the blackouts. Thus, the actors say their lines, there is a blackout and you can vaguely get a sense that the terps are still working! The interpreters are the stars of any ASL show and things must be set so they can do their job and be seen.

We have never had an ASL interpreted show without at least one full rehearsal with the terps onstage with the actors. Even just one run-through can be enough in a pinch for standard interpreting (supplemented with a director meeting with the terps to clarify text and meaning issues), but do that one run-through so all the actors onstage get used to the signing and do not watch it themselves. (ASL is a beautiful language and, for those not acquainted with it, it has a mesmerizing quality and a few times we have had child actors and adults alike start to watch the interpreters instead of paying attention to the onstage action.)

Do not make the mistake of performing a show featuring disabled performers without making provisions for the disabled audiences who will attend it. It does no good to present a play for disabled audiences that the disabled audience cannot see and experience. Do not present *Wait Until Dark*, a play about a young blind woman, without making provisions for blind audiences to attend and have a tactile tour of the set beforehand. Use things like D-Scriptive (an audio descriptive service) services or another program like closed captioning for performance narration if you have the funds and test it each night. Be very attentive that you do not negate the very work you are creating by not welcoming in the audiences you need. For those of us working in disability and inclusive theatre it is just as important to serve the disabled audiences as well as the artists. You are creating, enhancing and supporting a new community, an inclusive one, and thus you must be attentive to your audiences, readers of reviews, awards judges and anyone else who comes into your orbit. Your show may, as some of ours have done, become a 'hot' one because of a new performance style or some societal norm you challenge onstage or just because the acting is fabulous, and if it does you must be fully prepared for the sheer diversity of audience needs as your audiences increase and you sell out or add more performances. Anticipate everything before it happens. Plan ahead.

If we want to include people with disabilities in our theatres, then we need to better understand them as audience members, the physical and personal barriers they encounter, the attitudes they face and other issues that prevent their full participation. You need to not only research, ask, listen and open your mind, you also need to reach out and invest in this community. In order to invest in your audiences in performance you can experiment with audio description, also called media narration, which is someone narrating what is happening onstage in real time for a group in the audience who are listening via headphones. This is yet another example of some of the adaptive technology out there, like D-Scriptive. It is an acquired skill to learn to use the proper words to express imagery and context, but a great option if you can afford the system and the staff training. Universities in particular with their large budgets and endowments should be focusing not only on using these systems, but training their students on how to operate them and verbalize for them. There are many other technologies including closed captioning, which is expensive but worth it if you can afford it. Closed captioning is not a substitute for ASL performances although it may be easier to get funding for. Even if you use closed captioning you should plan for ASL work to be done. Closed captioning is a useful service for the hard of hearing or Deaf community. ASL, on the other hand, is a language and our investment in it as a company has been in an effort to join with the Deaf community in supporting and preserving this language.

As a policy, during your run you should always have backup plans for disabled artists if they need to travel to the theatre in bad weather. (Can they get in earlier to the theatre that day if needed to be sure to get in at all?) Remember accessible theory, or at least the version of accessible theory that I am proposing. Make all things work for all artists all the time. Universal accessibility. Equity. Have many secondary transportation options. Have enough trained staff to really welcome and deal with your varied audience members and their needs. Remember to have front of house and dressing room support as well as backstage support if your technical crew or staff is disabled and needs assistance.

In regard to disabled and non-disabled audience members during your performance run, you should use sensory guides with notes in your programs as to any triggers in the show and when they occur (which act, or which scene or even after which line). Loud noises can set off hyperacusis (a sensitivity to sound), as well as any odd smells and any use of fog or strobe lights. These triggers (similar to trauma triggers) can cause sometimes very emotional and disruptive reactions in your audience so know what some of the most basic triggers are and make provisions in case someone is triggered. Those in the audience with autism, cognitive and sensory disorders can benefit from knowing the possible triggers beforehand, as many times if they know it is coming they can deal with it and process it.

Again, have large-type programs for sight-impaired audience members or audience notices in the lobby of anything else you think may be pertinent (loud musical numbers, cast changes). Always err on the side of too much information. Be certain to add into PR and advertisements the dates of any ASL shows and the times for pre-show set tactile tours for the blind patrons if needed and do these tours after the actors need the stage for last warm up or any fight calls, musical numbers, etc. The tactile tours coming right before the house opens allows the actors their needed time in the space and also lets the tactile tour be very fresh in the disabled audience member's mind when the show begins shortly thereafter.

Once you are in the midst of the run and your artists and crew settle in, be sure to remain focused on the audience in performance. Have a TDD/TTY line for deaf patrons to call for ticket information (and this should be something that can be called at any time during your season, not just when tickets are on sale). Have active website links for all ticketing as well so contact can be made at all times. Have a text line and phone line free for the public to contact you and make certain your company has at least one public email contact, if not two or three. Group sales are often negotiated by phone so be certain they can contact you. Often we will send special invitations to schools, community groups, embassies, disability centers, veterans' groups, senior homes and groups, elected officials, specific community groups who serve immigrants or anyone we think will enjoy a certain production. We make certain we are reachable by all those whom we invite. You would be amazed what a personalized invitation can do for someone. We have had diplomats in our audiences, why? Because we invite them. Invite your board, donors, funders, make the effort to create a community around your work.

Continue to add in accessible technologies in performance not only for the performers but for the audience. Programs can be done in large print (remember the eighteen-point font minimum rule) and/or braille print (with a two-week request time if you are in a large city); if you use any assistive listening devices make sure they are checked each and every night as any technical things should be a part of the pre-show technical check list (this would also include electric wheelchair batteries being charged); always re-check all accessible entrances, backstage and restrooms in case something is blocking any of them. In cities where you need a licensed fire guard make sure you have two on staff at all times and be sure all exits are always clear. Have built into your fire evacuation plan all the needed provisions for patrons and artists in wheelchairs or with service dogs who may need mobility assistance as well as anyone needing visual assistance.

If you have audience attending with service dogs they will almost always let you know in advance, or your actors will know they are coming. If you can keep a few mats or blankets in the theatre for service dogs, do so. We also make sure to remove a seat in the audience so the service dog does not sit in, and block, the aisle. Instead, they get to be next to their person and out of harm's way. These service dogs deserve all the respect we can give them as they are on duty 24/7 taking care of someone and literally often being that person's lifeline out into the world.

We also try to save two empty spaces for each wheelchair user just to be sure they have room. Larger racing chairs or older electric chairs need extra room so we always make sure that is set. If they do not need the extra room, you just put the extra seat back into the audience. With a full range of openly sensory-friendly performances, and removable seating or even a row or two which can be removed or rearranged, you will have designed a space that creates a performing arts experience that is welcoming to all groups. We have even sat our audience members on couches and on bean bag chairs once.

Those companies which are actively doing children's shows (and it is vital you continue to do this and encourage our young disabled artists), just like with adults you could structure the shows to all of the awarenesses above and also to young audience members with autism or with other disabilities that create sensory sensitivities. Accommodations for all these needs could also include lowered sound levels, especially for startling or loud sounds or music. You can let house lights remain on at a low level in the theatre during the performance (just as you would with ASL shows), you can reduce or eliminate any strobe lighting or even temper the lighting focused or spilling out onto the audience.

You can even allow patrons the freedom to talk and leave their seats during the performance if they feel a bit overwhelmed. You can then designate quiet areas within the theatre lobby for them to sit. We have had times where we have had open space throughout parts of the theatre for standing and movement by the audience members who need it. If you have a show or can create a show that is free flowing enough to allow for this then do, even if only now and then. It is a great experience for everyone and especially for the younger audiences it really may be the difference between them attending or not. Even if you only do one sensory aware piece every two years it is still vital that you do it. There are so few sensory aware performances happening in any city that it is important that these audiences attend, and important that they see people like themselves onstage. They must have places of safety where they can see themselves reflected to the world.

On the last night of your performance run, whether you are going on to a local tour, a regional tour or ending the show entirely you will have your strike, or load-out. *Everyone* is part of our strikes, so sit down with your staff before the strike and pick specific tasks for each performer and crew member. Nobody gets out of the strike in our company, but each person has their job so that the strike becomes the last important component of the shared group experience. Try to match the ability and physicality with the strike component.

For example, if you have a little person in your cast, as we often do, we do not have them taking down lights (unless they want to), we have them doing something nearer to waist height so we do not risk their life, but we still get the work done. Artists with wheelchairs are great at being loaded up with things and then zipping costumes or props off to where they need to go. For those who need to be stationary they can remove gels from lights, fold costumes or wrap tieline, cut pizza, set up munchies, etc. This, of course, is what we plan, but very often we do have little people taking down lights and folks in wheelchairs dismantling flats. Whatever talent lends itself to best, whatever works for them and is safe, is what works for us.

Case Study 11: A Blind Actor and Discovering Colors,
Nicu's Spoon Theater, New York City

History

In around our 2007–2008 season we did a workshop of a new play, and I cast the leading role with a blind actor. The role was not written for a blind actor, however I chose to cast it as such. This was a deliberate casting choice geared toward a very wonderful actor. By this point our company was beginning to be known for our artistic choices and diversity and exploration of creative casting.

At a somewhat pivotal point in this production of the reading the leading actor had a lengthy monologue about a sunset. This was only a semi-staged workshop reading and no major physical movement was required so that the actor was able to read from his braille reader. However, I had chosen a wonderful blind actor to talk about colors for nearly three-quarters of a page. Granted, this was something that both he and I had known from the start and as we worked with the text it did become a bit apparent that his not having a background of identifying colors (he had been born blind and so had never identified colors) kind of 'un-colored' the speech.

Plan

What to do? This was not a panicked, last minute issue nor was it vital to the success of the piece, but it was something we both wanted to be right. So, what did we do?

See Chapter 16 for further details of this case study.

Chapter Action: The Strike Worklist and Delegating

So, here is your task. Using the same actors as listed in the chapter action for Chapter 7, about creating a period dance, and adding in a lighting tech person, a stage manager and an ASM and a director, make a full end-of-show strike checklist for a show of your choosing and designate who does what in the most logical way. In addition include all the socialization aspects, such as food and drink, gifts, speeches and so forth as we are assuming a cast party of sorts to go along with the strike. Examples of this will be on the companion website.

12

TECHNICAL CREW AND
TECHNICAL DESIGNS

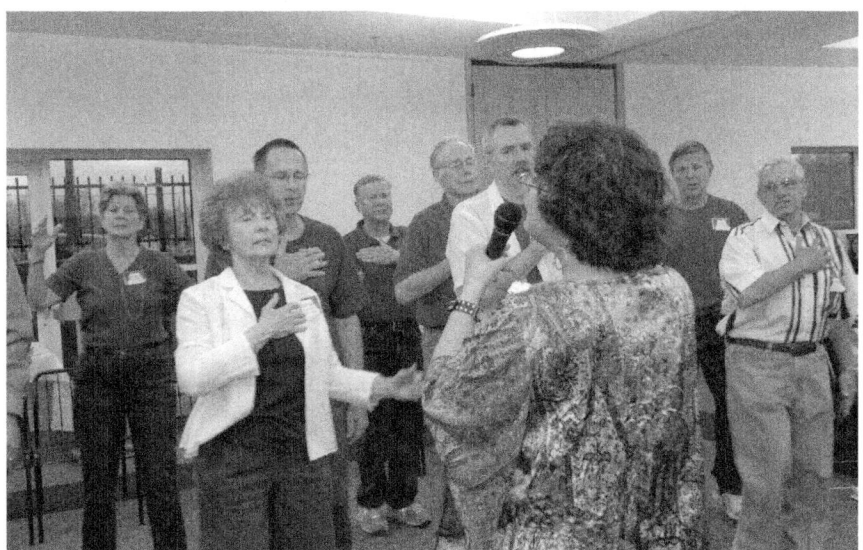

Figure 12.1 Joan Lipkin, of That Uppity Theatre Company, directs the Think Tank Performers. (Photograph courtesy of Marian Brickner.)

Darren Frazier, one of the signing members of the company and a veteran deaf sign-language actor, announced, "This was a new experience for me, groundbreaking." Kate Breen, who's also been signing ASL onstage for years, agreed, "This was intense."

United Stages, 'Stumps Innovative Double Casting'
by Maggie Cino, 2005

Your technical, design staff and stage crew are vital to any production and all of the above staff should have as much attendance as is possible during your production meetings and rehearsals. Not only can they see the process and have new ideas or become inspired, they must see the differing needs they will design for. Your design and technical staff can also stop you as producer or director from getting too 'inspired' with staging something they cannot possibly light or create due to budgets or time constraints. If your staff has disabilities you must begin to see how to take advantage of the new ways this may be creative for your production. As you accommodate them, pay attention to what other options it opens up for your show. Maybe you re-wire the light board so that you can move it to where they need it to be and it gives you a whole new angle on your perception of the stage so you end up staging the entire production differently. Perhaps you hire a color-blind lighting designer and see what that visual perception adds to the show. Some new designer may have an idea for a costume which needs to be big to fit around a wheelchair and that may then prompt you to all work out an entirely different entrance, ramp, archway or curtaining drape to get the actor onstage while wearing it. Having a staff member with a disability will change things from the ground up in planning your season and dealing with rehearsals. Always have at least one full production meeting per week during rehearsals with all designers, staff, volunteers and interns present. Since we are in a digital age now it is also easy to email and text ideas and pictures to each other as well as to have an online worksite/sharing place for ideas like basecamp.com or similar online meeting places.

Have your production staff challenge each other to find new ways to use all aspects of enhancements to complement artists with disabilities in your show such as ASL and captioning, anime and cartoons, multimedia, puppets that are either handheld or full body size, music of all kinds, dance and movement of all kinds, mime, singing in groups or solo and utilizing different languages (I think we have had fifteen languages spoken in our shows over the years), lighting or lack of lighting or different ways to light, sets with suspended portions, ramps, too many stairs, not enough stairs, play with all of it. Experimentation should be utilized not as a vague concept or something you do in an emergency, but as a stand-alone production tool so you can actively work on training new crew, young directors and new artists with disabilities as well as expanding the minds of young new non-disabled designers.

I have worked with many young stage managers and designers right out of some of the best theatrical college training programs in the US and as of yet, unless they have a disability themselves (or know someone who does), they have very little idea about what the ADA is, how to work with or stage disabled artists or what any of the options are for themselves in designing or working with disabled artists in full-scale productions. These new graduates also assume that in the real world they will have access to a full costume build shop (like in college), a full 'shop' and building dock location (like in college) and a fairly unlimited supply of funding (like in college). None of this prepares them to produce on shoestring budgets (or any budgets really) at times or to creatively problem solve in regional theatres or smaller houses. For this, I fault the universities that train these young people but do not prepare them for the real world of work in even regional theatres which have strict budgets. I liken it to graduating from an acting program, filled with prestige and promise, and yet having absolutely no idea how to present yourself in a real-life professional audition situation. Prosaic though the idea may seem, graduating theatre majors must be better prepared to work and create in the real world.

If you have a stage manager with a disability, the one main issue for you will be that if they are a wheelchair user they cannot lug tons of things around on their lap or in their arms so you need an ASM who can. I have not yet met nor heard of a stage manager who is blind, although I know of two who are deaf (in which case I would have at least one ASL speaking ASM). If you do have a stage manager in a wheelchair or with a major mobility issue, and the cast size is over twelve, then have two ASMs. If your stage manager is blind or deaf then have a sighted assistant or a hearing assistant who can sign. It is about the balance of talents.

If you are like my company and other inclusive companies, you will have had some long-term staff members who are not only incredible human beings, but fearless talented artists and people who are accepting of all types of inclusion, even if they are non-disabled. My long-term lighting designer, Steven Wolf, started when we began the company in 2001 and eventually became my Associate Artistic Director and my touchstone as to what we could or could not do, "Steph, we can't simultaneously fly four actors in wheelchairs over the stage on a $500 budget" he would say calmly, shaking his head. No matter the technical problem he takes a deep breath and works to solve it.

Likewise, our company composer Damon Law, has grown with us since 2001 and has even composed music for shows with specific body types, nationalities, mobilities and disabilities in his head as he works. Pamela Mitchell has been with us since 2003 and has helped to create our ASL programs and projects, joined by Bram Weiser in 2005. They have all, as have many others, shaped our work and been co-brains in many of our creative projects. They all have an inherent personal acceptance and love of others that is as important to me in working with them as their talent is.

You and your staff of designers and running crew also have to have many brains to think of ways of creative problem solving. Most light booths are high up and overlook the stage so you can either have a sled (really like a small sled or backboard made of wood which someone is strapped to and then slowly whisked up the stairs into the booth, but only if they do not have spinal issues) to get your crew up into the booth or move and rewire the booth equipment (the lightboard and sound mixer, etc.) to a ground floor location with good stage sightlines for the run of your show.

Somewhere, someday, someone will design a light booth which hydraulically lowers onto the ground and then the crew can get in, wheelchairs and all or accommodating any kind of disability. Then the light booth can be hydraulically lifted back up into whatever high place it needs to be. This, of course, doesn't solve bathroom breaks during intermission without lowering the whole thing (unless there is a bathroom in the light booth itself), but one step at a time…

Case Study 12: That Uppity Theatre Company

St Louis, Missouri, Joan Lipkin
Producing Artistic Director

History

Our name reflects who we are. Bold, brave, willing to step outside the status quo in order to instigate social change, promote civic dialogue and produce transformative theatrical art of the highest quality for people of all ages. Like most groundbreaking endeavors, we don't fit very well into a neat category of description. Sometimes, we perform in gymnasiums, other times in corporate board rooms. We have even performed in a car wash.

Since we began in 1989, our work has taken many forms in response to the needs of the times. Currently, we often create commissioned work about social issues for corporations, schools from elementary through university-level and social services agencies. In other ongoing projects, we also pair amateur actors and seasoned professionals to create work about the lives of underrepresented populations. We have also increasingly focused on workshops that promote the development of empathy and emotional intelligence through performance techniques.

For our 'Think Tank' project, I was approached by the Alzheimer's Association about running a potential theatre class for people with dementia and early-stage Alzheimer's. One of the staff members of the Alzheimer's Association knew of my work with different populations including blind youth, LGBTQIA youth and adults and women with cancer as well as our ongoing work with people with disabilities. She thought it would be a good fit and an interesting opportunity to expand the programming being offered to the people the association served.

I believe deeply in the creative capacity of all people and of the life enhancing possibilities of arts activities, especially performance, so it was a challenge that I was excited to take on. Additionally, I have a personal connection to Alzheimer's, as my late aunt was diagnosed with Alzheimer's and I watched her family struggle to provide quality care for her.

Interestingly, only two of the people in the class were female. Everyone else was male. And the ages ran from early fifties to mid seventies. Initially, my activities were designed to ascertain the interests, backgrounds and attention capacity of the various members of the group. No one in the St Louis area had done this kind of work before and I only knew of one other group nationally that was working with people with memory loss so there was no roadmap for us to follow.

Our theatre company is a registered internship and practicum site for social work students. Given the complexity of the project and the participants, I decided to invite students with a particular interest in gerontology to work along with us for additional support and to provide them with a unique learning opportunity.

When we first started, I used conversation circles as a way to gather initial information about the background of individuals in the group, but it was challenging for them to sustain interest in hearing what each other had to say in that configuration for any sustained period of time. Often, their interest would flag or they would become distracted or preoccupied with their own thoughts. So focusing on narrative or linear structure was less productive.

But they loved music, so I would play music from different eras and often, they sang along and I encouraged dancing. One very interesting by-product of Alzheimer's and early-stage dementia is that certain inhibitions as well as social mores seem to drop away. Heterosexual men would happily dance, partnered together. They were also very open to doing improvisation, especially if it used movement and I suggested specific characters for them to play.

One day, I suggested that we stage the Lewis and Clark expedition. We discussed what elements were needed for a trip down the river. We determined that we needed Lewis as well as Clark but I was surprised when someone said, "What about the little dog? We need a little dog for the boat." Apparently, somewhere in the reaches of this man's mind, he must have recalled a painting of the Lewis and Clark expedition with a little dog at the bow.

Sometimes I would lead them towards responses through questions they could be successful answering. I said, "So we are in a boat. Shall we all row together?" And I introduced a movement with which they could then work. I might begin to narrate the story by saying, "The wind is whipping up. Can you feel the wind?" I might become the wind and most of them would happily follow and embellish on their own if I provided a physicalized example using movement and making sound effects. We traveled all the way down the river this way, encountering storms and wild animals. We played. It was great fun.

Plan

If one thinks in traditional performance terms, the greatest challenge might have been the inability to memorize lines or retain blocking. The Alzheimer's Association charged me with both running a weekly class as well as creating a final performance for caregivers and family members. But I have always thought outside the box when it comes to working with and for marginalized populations. And I define performance as a series of conscious moments for a designated audience. There is tremendous latitude within that concept.

What difference would it make if our social work students or I also acted as side coaches to provide support or structure during the performance so that the participants could feel safe? It made it no less a performance, according to my definition. And arguably, it was useful because it made clear the structures we chose in order to best support our participants.

So that is what we did. We entered improvisationally, dancing through a room of about 300 people to *I Heard it Through the Grapevine*. I explained to the audience that we were the Think Tank Players and had a wonderful performance for them in which we would all take part.

See Chapter 16 for further details of this case study.

13

ACADEMIC TRAINING ASSESSMENT AND SUSTAINABILITY

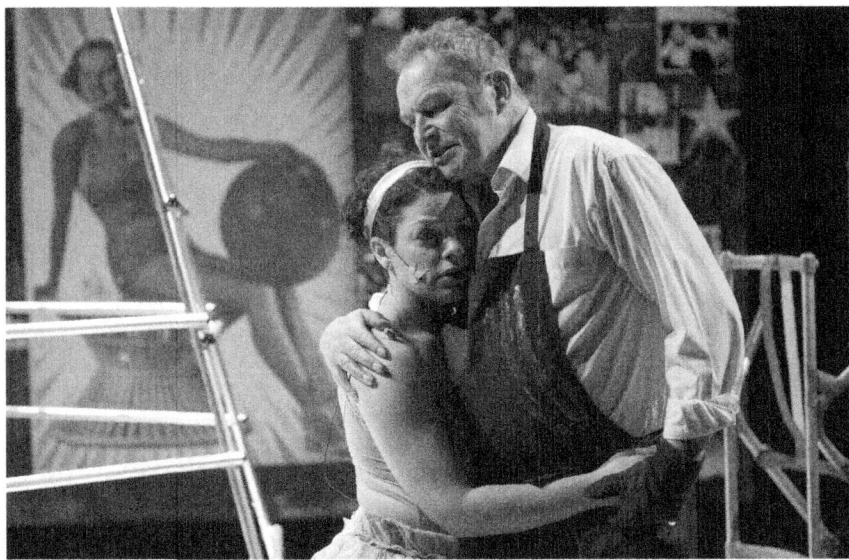

Figure 13.1 Raspberry, UK Tour 2010 co-production of Fittings Multimedia Arts and Sounds of Progress. Written by Garry Robson, Christine Bruno and Jem Dobbs. (Photograph courtesy of Tim Morozzo.)

I am challenging the following colleges and universities—Brown University, Yale University, NYU, the Juilliard School, Florida State University, the University of Minnesota, the University of Iowa, the University of Texas, the University of Washington, University of California—Berkeley, Stanford University, and California Institute of the Arts—to come together and form a consortium dedicated to identifying and developing disabled theatre artists with the goal of creating a new generation of leaders of the American theatre. As some of the colleges and universities with the largest endowments in the country will be involved in this project, it is not a question of finances. It is a question of desire and value.

Brad Rothbart, *American Theatre Magazine*, October 2015, 'Once More Unto the Breach: An Anatomized Philippic Regarding the Relationship of Disability to the Contemporary American Theatre'

As I write this book in June 2016, the University of Kentucky has created a Universal Design program dedicated to creating and building accessible spaces, and there is a new Universal Design in Education Training Team for faculty and instructors at the University of Oregon. Universal design is not synonymous with accessibility, as universal design has at its core a leveling of the playing field effect where the ultimate design serves the populace as a whole, disabled and non-disabled. This is heartening news at a time when Hollywood still dismays us all by releasing the film *Me Before You*, an ode to life being worthless once you become disabled and so you should leave your money to someone who can enjoy life and then kill yourself. The growing vocal, political and articulate disability community is now finding that it can seriously damage box office for a major motion picture like this one as well as generate positive PR for a university. This is a very different power than this community had twenty years ago. The twenty-first century disabled artistic community is growing in power and will soon be a political force larger than they have ever been (one in six voters has a disability, keep in mind) and they will continue to demand training, promotion, equitable casting and pay and substantial work. The universities that are smart enough to get it together now and start training artists with disabilities will be on the front lines of the changing theatre, television and film scene in the US.

A special note for disabled students reading this. You have the right to ask for and expect full accessibility into your classes, restrooms, dorm rooms, lecture halls, cafeterias, rehearsal rooms, backstage, dressing rooms, onstage, in the booth, any place on the campus or that caters to the campus must be accessible for you. You have the right to demand that. If you are shy then contact your disability office on campus and ask them for support. You have the right to have classroom notetakers available if you cannot take notes. You have the right to record your classes, or have them recorded for you if needed. You have the right to refer your university to www.assistivetech.net or any other website which can provide them with information and technology they can utilize in order to make you comfortable in your studies. This is the law. You are not required to be an ambassador for your disability unless you wish to be and you do not have to be diplomatic and not ask for what you need. You are not required to 'settle' for sitting outside a classroom, listening, because you cannot get in the door. Do ask for what you need. You cannot receive the full benefit of an education if you cannot go to all of the places that you need to go.

An institution of higher learning cannot even begin to address the issue of sustaining what they are doing financially, internally or academically until it has done an assessment of where it is and what it is currently doing. It is not up to students with disabilities to have to fight for access and training any longer, although chronically this is how it has been in the past. It is up to the universities to provide this to them from day one. This must cease to be something students must become activists and advocates to achieve. Universities usually are self-sustaining, they just must adjust to putting disability studies, services and theatre practicum into their curriculum and daily life. Universities have many resources at their disposal to do this and the funding is there on a federal level, so universities must get off their … podiums … and get to work.

Even a basic assessment of your university must address issues such as student access and accessibility feedback (have you requested feedback from your students who are disabled?), enforcement of state and federal accessibility laws, audience and community turn-out at events (and their feedback), transportation to and from housing for your students with disabilities, the exploration of adjusted training methods to support varied students and the evolution of your continued work on the curriculum. Existing accommodations and technology, questionnaires, online surveys, increases in website hits, a simple tour around every inch of your campus with someone in a wheelchair and someone who is blind will provide a wealth of information on what does not work and what does. Contact me or one of the many people I mention in this book and ask them to walk your campus or to set up an action plan for your university. Ask them to do staff training in vocabulary and awareness.

Your mailing list growth and requests for information are all assessment indicators that can be quantified to see if what you are doing is right and may even be further sustainable. Good assessment figures also help when speaking to the government, board members, elected officials, foundations and individual donors about their assistance in sustaining your institution or beginning new programs for students with disabilities, or even just adding new technologies they can utilize. A university endowment campaign should not, in my opinion, even be started unless there are full provisions for disabled students, curriculum, training, resources and placement in said university and in said campaign.

Academics and college level inclusion is woefully not only usually inactive, but inadequate. Why there is not a major university in the US (admittedly there is Gallaudet University, but that is primarily for deaf students in dance and acting) that is fully physically accessible that is also *actively* recruiting and training disabled actors, directors, playwrights, arts facility managers, designers, stage managers, set and lighting designers, fight choreographers, producers and musical directors I have no idea. If I could build a university or if someone hired me to run a theatre department, I would put this into practice immediately.

The auditioning boards of major arts universities need to be deliberately created who are able to address not only the active recruitment of disabled students, but also to assess any training and/ or class adjustments that need to be made upon their acceptance. Putting an artist with a disability on your auditioning board is a brilliant (and realistic) move. This practice, if put into place, would literally start to change the face of theatre education in the US. It increases profits for the university as well and again you can get federal funds to add, adjust or make accessible any area on your campus. The money is there for the taking if you have the proper plans to apply for it.

That aside, every theatre department and theatre major course of study in the US should have at least one course of an inclusive theatre practicum, complete with vocabulary and history discussions. Every graduating director should feel ready to direct a disabled actor or a disabled cast by the time he or she gets their degree. Every non-disabled artist should be ready to work with a disabled counterpart. Every set designer should know how to build an ADA compliant ramp (and most do not) and how to think outside the box in designing a universal design set. Every drama or performance or theatre program should do a play about disability once a season and plot out their curriculum to support this. It is not up to students to ask for it, nag about it and demand it any longer. Playwrights should be actively grown from the disabled community as well and no academic programs have even woken up to this. All academic recruiters should be actively looking at disabled students. Let me say again, *twenty percent*. *One-fifth* of the United States has a disability and there is not one American university dedicated to training them in the performing arts. This is a glaring error.

Granted, most universities have a disabilities office, disability program or disability coordinator, but these are primarily for housing assistance, transportation assistance and benefit assistance. Usually these offices are themselves often run by non-disabled people who do not understand why disabled students cannot be 'satisfied' with this or that issue. These offices are about 'satisfying' a momentary issue, but more is needed. You wouldn't ask a non-disabled student to be 'satisfied' with watching a class on film instead of live because you cannot get them into the classroom, why would you ask the same (yet charge the exact same amount of money for tuition) from a disabled student? You would not tell a non-disabled student that he or she should be lucky the one bus they can take to school stops for them three hours before they need to be in class, why then would you expect a disabled student to take that bus and then sit for three hours outside before class begins? There are even, unbelievably, disability offices in a few American universities which do not have a ramp for wheelchair access into them and rarely is there a disability services office which has an employee who is disabled on staff. There must be change at a very basic level in university disability services.

Moreover, nobody in these disabilities offices is teaching artists with disabilities the practical job know-how of how to design lights or direct a show or run a sound mixer (or, come to think of it, run a theatre company as a business). Not one of these disability offices is encouraging a young disabled playwright, director, composer or set designer. This is beyond neglectful, beyond even the mandates of most universities and it must change. It will change. The change is coming. The choice is to be on board, or not, with that change.

Universities must keep up with the rest of the world by preparing their own staff, board and directors to be inclusive. Why ignore twenty percent of the population that you could be training and working with? If for no other reason than just to make money off of that twenty percent, someone should be looking very carefully at their recruiting and curriculum. I hate to appeal to the inherent greed that abounds, but if it gets a university program moving to develop a theatre training program for disabled students, I'll take it. If greed motivates a university dean to start to be inclusive, then let's start with that.

A beautiful place to start for any university is adding a board member who is disabled, or a performing arts teacher or an auditioner. Another step could be something technical such as the elimination of light booths above the stage or the creation of a light booth built on a crane or hydraulic lift mentioned earlier. My alma mater, California Institute of the Arts, has great potential in something like their hydraulically-run modular theatre. The modular theatre is built of 4 × 6 foot wide platforms, each operated by a hydraulic lift, that can be raised and lowered to configure any stage at all, even a flat one. The Fei & Milton Wong Experimental Theatre at SFU Woodward's in Vancouver, BC has also been seen as a beacon in the theatrical accessibility venue arena.

This accessibility and inclusion also pertains to young architects and the construction of new buildings and arts complexes with full universal design and access features. Architecture students should have universal design courses and disability studies as part of their normal curriculum, not something that is a specialty item or an optional elective. How can we work with these artists with disabilities if the buildings are not being built for us to *all* be in together? How can any of this theatre be done unless the audiences, all types of audiences, can get into the space comfortably to see the work?

This societal attitudinal perception that you do have control over (addressed in Chapter 10) in your press and external relations is even more important for universities and recruiters or speakers in academia to understand and to utilize. A university discussing the new Disabilities Services office or position with a faint tone of distaste or pity is not the way to go. Announcing it proudly and with excitement (online, in person, on your website, in interviews) is much better because it *is* exciting to be creating and filling these new positions so you can then serve the new disabled students, whom you will soon begin to recruit, better. Universities must begin to see the potential and get excited about the changes working with these artists will bring.

Any university should also ensure that students with disabilities have their health care needs met. This may sound off subject and somewhat out of the blue, however, disabled students at times cannot access health care facilities on campus and in some cases females with disabilities have found increased problems with even getting birth control, either because the health center is not accessible or because their need for it is treated like a dirty joke. Both of these issues impact health and artistic access. Artistic access is only part of the iceberg needing to be melted. "If a culture's language is full of pejorative metaphors about a group of people," writer and artist with late-diagnosed autism, Rachel Cohen-Rottenberg, wrote in a 2013 *Disability and Representation* article, "that culture is more likely to view those individuals as less entitled to rights like housing, employment, medical care, education, access, and inclusion." Add to that list the political and societal perception that disabled people are less entitled to love, sexual activity and parenting and you are closer to the mark.

Full inclusion in universities leaves no room at all for treating anyone's health needs as if they are not important or as something that they should have to fight for. Healthy students are what you want. Not some who are healthy and some who are not, some who go to class and some who sit outside, some who can access classes and some who have to 'figure it out' or 'make do with it,' some who are treated as human beings and some who are excluded from all decent rights and treatment. Inclusion means we all get in, we all have class, we all access everything, we all are healthy and treated with respect.

A challenge was issued in the November 2015 issue of *American Theatre Magazine* and is reprinted as a quote at the start of this chapter. How many universities will accept Brad Rothbart's challenge?

Case Study 13: The Glass Menagerie, *an Actor's Personal Case Study*

Christine Bruno, New York City

History

Laura, like most disabled characters, has traditionally been viewed through a non-disabled lens; definitely by non-disabled people, but I would argue, by most disabled people as well. In some ways, disabled people have been even more guilty of accepting Laura's pitiable narrative than many of our non-disabled counterparts, if for no other reason than to rally against it. I know I was.

I actively rebelled against stepping into Laura's shoes for more than a decade. Disabled since birth and armed with the knowledge since age five that I wanted to be an actor, I thumbed my nose at the presumption by nearly every person, industry professional or layperson who'd read or seen the play, that I was *born* to play Laura. How could I possibly play Laura? I was nothing like her. She's a weak, shrinking violet plagued by insecurity and trapped between her mother's disappointment, delusions and unrealistic expectations for her children. I am an incisive, opinionated conversationalist with a strong sense of self, a healthy sexual appetite, and an innate desire to shatter with impunity any assumption or boundary that finds its way into my path. I wasn't going to wipe out a lifetime of internal activism to be some director's token 'cripple,' so that they could pat themselves on the back for a bold and risky casting choice and the audience could bask in their superiority of simultaneous pity and 'there but for the grace of God go I' mentality.

Even though I loved the play and had worked on it in acting classes more than once over the years, I clung to that 'badge of honor,' which, in retrospect, I attribute to equal parts lack of maturity and a refusal to embrace my identity as a disabled person versus a person with a disability.

So, when the opportunity to play Laura presented itself in September 2001, I was incredibly conflicted, but 'Blue Roses' (Jim calls Laura 'Blue Roses,' a mispronunciation of pleurosis, the childhood disease that left Laura with a limp) was impossible to ignore. I wish I could take credit for the serendipitous wisdom of that decision, but the truth is, I wanted, needed and as it turned out, was willing to fight for the job.

Plan

When word got out that a well-respected regional theatre on the east coast was holding auditions, at least a dozen friends sent the notice my way, in case I hadn't been paying attention. I had and had already contacted my agent, with whom I had signed less than a month before, about getting me an appointment. After a week, I had heard nothing and the audition was less than a week away, I paid my agent a visit. He told me he had contacted the casting director and her response was, "I don't think the director would be interested in seeing an actor with a disability for this role." I replied with a shocked laugh, "has she read the play?!" But I knew it wasn't a joke. I also knew it was going to be up to me to fight for the opportunity to be seen.

I had an uncomfortable conversation with my agent when I mentioned it was illegal for the casting director to deny me an audition based on my disability. He told me in no uncertain terms that it would do neither one of us any good for him to jeopardize his relationship with this prominent casting director. Luckily, with the help of his assistant, I was able to convince him that I was in fact 'perfect' for the role (to my shock, he had never read the play!) and he agreed to go over the casting director's head and call the director because he had a client in the show currently running at the theatre. His call to the director was brief. "I have a client who is perfect for the role of Laura. She has a physical disability. Would you be willing to see her?" – "Of course!" I was in!

Now came the hard part: preparing for the audition.

See Chapter 16 for further details of this case study.

How Well Is Your Institution Doing?

This chapter is for the academics, teachers and board members reading this. You are intelligent and presumably good at what you do so put your head into any disabled person's so you can pre-understand their needs. Take a walk around your campus, invite someone with a disability to come with you. Is your campus even ADA compliant at all? If it, or any aspect of it, was built after 1992 then it must be ADA compliant or compliant with the Uniform Federal Accessibility Standards (UFAS). Keep in mind that your building being up to local building standards may not make it ADA and federally compliant. Can the students get from the bus stop into their classes? Look at your course offerings, are they fully inclusive? Are they worded in inclusive language? Is there anything at all in your PR materials that encourages and welcomes disabled students? Do you employ assistive listening devices? Are your recruiters targeting disabled students? Do you have materials printed in braille and/or large font printing? Is your audition board prepared to audition them in a fully accessible space and then make any adjustments needed for their full education in the arts? Does your website 'speak' to a blind applicant? Do your elected officials, both on a local and state level, have discretionary funds which can assist you? "Maybe, but," you think, "we can't just say we welcome disabled arts students, please apply!"

Why not? Why can't you? That is precisely what you can and need to do. You must invite them in. This is a populace that has spent their lives being deliberately excluded and now if need be, they must be deliberately included. If you really feel you can't state or publicize an invitation, then what can you do to change your own perception? How can you change your recruitment officials, materials or where and how you do recruitment fairs? Map out five ideas that your university could change immediately to actively recruit, audition and train disabled artists. Map out how to audition and accommodate them fully. Have your development office look into the federal programs and monies available to create, rebuild, develop and sustain new programming for the disabled. Hire a consultant to come in and revamp what you are doing, look at your spaces, and suggest ten steps to take. Heck, call me and I will do it for you. More information and resources for this can be found on the companion website.

14

ASSESSMENT AND SUSTAINABILITY IN THEATRES

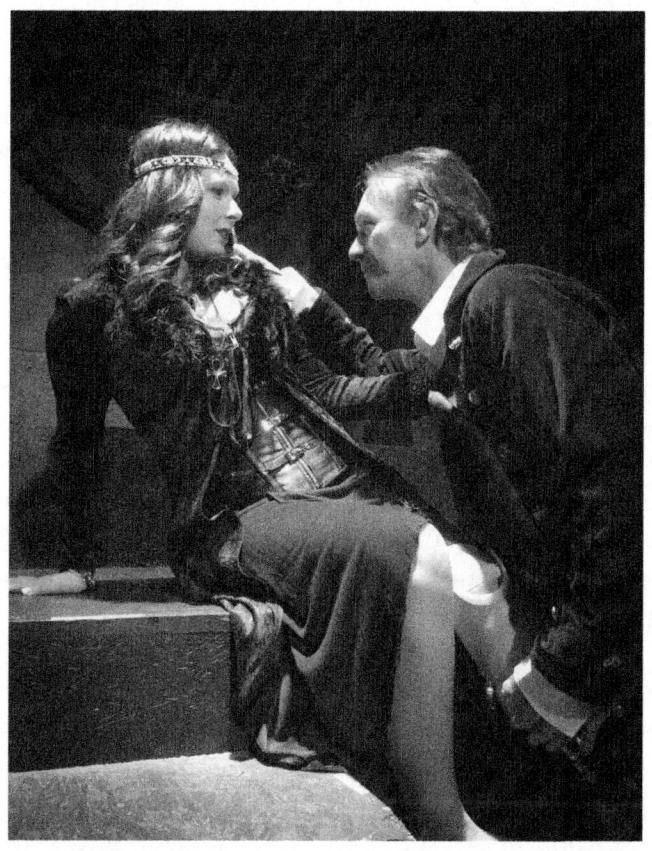

Figure 14.1 Richard III by William Shakespeare, 2015. L to R Rachel Handler and Guy Ventoliere. (Photograph courtesy of Damon Law.)

It's math time, folks. Visibly physically disabled people (not counting the blind or deaf) make up 10 percent of the population. There are approximately 50 major resident theatres in the U.S. that pay a full-time living wage and benefits. Those theatres have an average of four people on their top artistic staff: an artistic director, an associate artistic director, a literary manager and a literary associate. That's $50 \times 4 = 200$. For visibly physically disabled people to have a representative voice in American resident theatres, there should be 20 employees who fit that description: five artistic directors, five associate artistic directors, five literary managers, and five literary associates... I have no doubt that the American resident theatres fails this test.

Brad Rothbart, *American Theatre Magazine,*
October 2015 'Once More Unto the Breach: An Anatomized
Philippic Regarding the Relationship of Disability to the
Contemporary American Theatre'

In the *American Theatre Magazine* issue of November 2015 they devoted the *whole* issue to disabilities and disabled artists. Well, let's be honest shall we? They put in *some* articles and gave the cover to *Spring Awakening* which the wonderful company Deaf West did on Broadway with disabled artists in it, but not really the whole issue. Again, this is pretty illustrative of the sheer scale of the problem. The premiere American magazine for theatre did some serious PR regarding the 'disability issue,' however maybe only one-half of the magazine had any actual disability issues in it. They did, to their credit, publish an utterly mesmerizing and brilliant essay by Brad Rothbart *Once More Unto the Breach: An Anatomized Philippic Regarding the Relationship of Disability to the Contemporary American Theatre,* probably the best and most honest writing I have ever read on the reality of disability in theatre, which is why you will find quotes from it in this book. But, in their 'Role Call,' the 'people to watch in theatre' section, not one person was disabled. Not a playwright, actor or director. Not a staff member of an inclusive company, not a disabled theatre professional at all.

In not one of the many ads in this magazine (present in every single issue throughout the year) about auditions at prestigious programs for artists, not one of them spotlighted and said "We are very proud to welcome artists with disabilities to audition." (In the disabled issue!!! Hello?) Well, you could say, it is implied. No. No, it isn't. It is not implied at all. Not ever. Not if you are an artist with a disability. Not if you want to be an artist and you just happen to be disabled. It is not implied at all, ever. Society doesn't imply it, history does not imply it, theatres do not and the schools and training programs do not either. That is why it must be said and said again. The invitation must be made (and it must be made publicly and repeatedly) by the programs, the universities, the recruiters and the local and regional theatres.

In assessing all levels of inclusion in the arts possibilities in the US there is no level in the theatrical world, the film and television world and the university world where we are not lacking. We do not want to train disabled artists or even really want to take them seriously as artists if truth be told. (Have you ever begged out of a performance of something featuring artists with disabilities because you just knew it would be awful?) Shame on you. Shame on us and our assumptions. Shame, as well, on theatre practitioners and companies which do work with artists who are disabled, but have their rehearsals closed to other theatre creators who would like to learn best practices from them. Shame on you for not sharing how you do what you do. Shame on you for not hiring interns and mentoring young directors. How can we grow this theatre if we do not share information, train interns and let people see what we do and how we do it? We must compete for funds, that is the nature of the beast, however, we can share our processes and best practices without rancor. Hopefully this book will get us all started.

There is a new term gaining ground in all rights groups, 'intersectionality,' which is where one or more marginalized points intersect in one person, one place or one issue. My company has been working in this area for years, calling it inclusion, and finally we have an 'official' term for it. An African-American lesbian who is an amputee, for instance, is a prime example of intersectionality. This intersectionality as it pertains to groups cannot be ignored as it is a huge part of our population and over time, as in the LGBTQIA community, it is becoming not only a force for social progress but also a powerful voting block. For heads of funding agencies, for casting directors, for political figures denying accessible funds I must tell you to get with the program because soon you will be voted out and replaced. The disability movement, and the intersectionality with other voting block groups, is becoming strong and theatre and art is one of the arenas where they have long been denied entry.

It does not matter what size and budget your organization is in order to do this work. Over our seventeen seasons our largest budgeted year was a tad under $250,000 and our lowest budgeted year was a bit over $15,000 for our first season. Sustainability is both about money and about structure, planning and long-term thinking. You can, as I have, produce with any amount of money, whether it be $50,000 or $5 billion. However, it is the long-term planning, donor cultivation, constant self-assessment, goals and vision you must utilize to grow. As of this writing there are funds at city, county, regional, state and federal levels in all fifty states of the US. If that should change (and even if it does not) and those funds are lacking, then that is where your community work and investment comes into play. People give money to things they are a part of and invested in. People invest in you by your investing in them.

Plan for the long haul. Evaluation is a roadmap of your trip. It helps you to connect the dots. If you do not have a code of ethics and a company policies document, get to work. Do you have an emergency preparedness plan? (It should include a section on what to do in a full audience situation and should cover any contingencies for company members and audience with disabilities. In New York after 9/11 you can bet everyone made emergency plans.) Do you have an ADA verification of compliance question set filled out? Do you have a policy of inclusion not only for your artists, but for your staff and board? You should. This shows long-term, serious planning. You can even plan long term with more politically risky contemporary 'freak show' productions which glorify and proudly work with disabled artists in owning their disabilities, their 'crip value.' However you must have serious long-term planning involved as well as a complete understanding of crip value and crip culture. Examples of planning for the long haul can be found on the companion website.

Those theatres that are lucky enough to own or lease their own theatre space also have a renting possibility they must cultivate. We leased our theatre for five years in midtown Manhattan and rather than deal with the wear and tear of constant short-term renters we developed our 'resident company' program where two to three superb companies were 'resident' in our space. They were guaranteed their season had a place to perform (a good thing in a quickly changing city like New York City) and they were given a cut in rental fees. We were guaranteed that like-minded and responsible companies (who also worked with diverse artists) were in our space when we were not actively using it. In addition, the wear and tear on the space itself was less, because it truly was their home as well as ours. This planning, as well as renting spaces out for classes and the like, illustrates thoughtful financial thinking.

In assessing your own company as an entity keep it very simple to start. What assets do you have? A theatre? Lights? Costume stock? Props? Weaponry? Do you have a public relations team or a staff photographer? In your company members do you have a choreographer? A music director? A fight director? A licensed fire marshal? A licensed electrician? (Assets are also people and talents.) What do you need? What audience issue, community issue or production problem do you see a need for? Do you need ramps or an assistive listening system? What goals do you set to solve this issue or to serve a certain audience? What are your objectives? What are your expected outcomes? What are your plans to measure these outcomes? (Income, audience attendance, grants gotten, for example. This must be quantifiable.) What are your expenses? Quantifiable information is the best gateway to sustainability as you must be able to plan for, track and account for every single thing you do or need.

Theatres today must also continue to assess their own energy and strength. Many theatres, especially those working outside the mainstream and with diverse artists, get so little support and work so hard (yet are not applying for grants) that they are endlessly exhausted and cannot even take the time to develop best practices, let alone share or teach them. For instance, nearly forty theatre companies across the US were contacted for input into this book and three-quarters of the theatres responded with excitement about how necessary it was and how much the information needed to be shared and disseminated into universities and other theatres, however they themselves were so overwhelmed with work that they felt they had nothing of value to contribute. I myself had to back out of producing with my company for six months to write this book so I understand the exhaustion. Luckily some of the very finest companies in the US did find the time to share their case studies and knowledge. My undying respect to them all in sharing what works and even more important, what did not work.

Do not let your theatre and your company develop a 'caregiver theatre' mentality where the work bogs down the energy of the company and its staff and any social, political, educational and online impact your group can have. You are not caregivers, and the artists with disabilities you work with do not need your 'care,' they need to work. Thus, a vital part of your assessment must be slowing down and realizing your own best practices and what works. Do not make the mistake of not sharing information and lessons with other groups or individuals. Information truly is power.

The state of theatre in the US has to change and your theatre can and should be at the forefront of it. We must collectively create a number of spaces that artists with disabilities want to be included in, create places they are asked to come, are invited into and feel safe in. Yes, this space should already be in existing schools and universities, in acting classes, in all auditions, in theatre companies, in all theatres, in all touring companies, on Broadway, in dramas and comedies and musicals, on television and in film and commercials and in children's shows. But it is not.

In the coming years more and more creative technology (now Waverly Labs has the Pilot, an earpiece that allows two people to converse, each in their own language, and it translates for them) will become available for theatre practitioners to use. Virtual reality training is now being used to help paraplegics move their limbs. There are experimental gloves now (invented by MIT undergraduate students Thomas Pryor and Navid Azodi) called SignAloud that translates some ASL signs into verbalized and audible speech. There are new form-fitted arm crutches which hold weight on the forearm and streamline how the body moves in using them. The change in the movement and kinesiology of the wearer of these crutches is breathtaking. There is a disabled engineer, Hugh Herr, who has created robotic legs which take their movement cues from the wearer's own nerves. There is Dr Josh Miele at Smith-Kettlewell Research Institute in San Francisco who has invented a new technology called WearaBraille, which is a virtual wireless braille keyboard with iPhone and voice over control. What you type or say is converted into braille immediately. We have no idea what is coming in the future in the way of technology (bionic eyes? walking wheelchairs?) but one thing I do know. All these creative technologies will increasingly bring disabled people together and out into the world and we have to be there to meet them.

There is a way to access these technologies as they become available, especially if you are a well-known regional theatre company or have a professional season. Be very specific about what you want and ask for it from the inventor or apply for it. Ask to use WearaBraille for a season, ask to have an artist use the streamlined crutches for a production. The important thing is to ASK. Many large theatres bemoan the lack of funding they get, however, when their grants or funding patterns are analyzed you discover they have applied for either no grants at all, very low-level funds or equipment that does not match their size or theatrical impact. Be very specific and realistic, "We want to fund three ASL performers and build four accessible wheelchair ramps this season." And approach the funders thusly. If you feel you are too close to the issues and cannot analyze your grant patterns, again contact one of the resources in this book and they can help you.

In addition, approach your board members time and time again. Boards must be vested in your theatre company and must give something every year whether it be money, time, connections to funders or individual donors or their manual labor. We have had years where one board member donated a large chunk of funds and another one sat and licked stamps and helped with box office. Both were wonderful and their contributions needed. It is not enough for them to sit on your board, make them do something. By doing something they have an implied ownership in the outcomes and successes of your company or your university.

Continually assessing what you do as a theatre company must also be priority. You must be able to not only know exactly what you do (and how to talk about it to others), illustrate how it should work, prove that it works, illustrate how you know that it works and show facts and figures to back that up, but also to keep up ongoing assessment activities which can turn not only individual donors, but foundations and perhaps even state or governmental donors into yearly funders. If your theatre does not track attendance numbers, mailing list growth, website hits, donor figures, feedback online and post-show (questionnaires and feedback slips are very useful) reactions from audience members (audience members at my shows all know I am there in the lobby and frequently tell me their opinions), staff and cast numbers, special projects, numbers of kids or community members served and more, you are wasting your time and energy. You must track all of this as well as unique visitors to your website, ticket sales figures, website hits per show, per activity, per day, per season of the year – literally anything that can be tracked, added up, analyzed, quantified and tallied should be. Only then can you begin to see the repeated patterns of growth which you can then use to approach donors with projects and events geared toward your sustainability.

Theatre companies that are producing toward sustainability and using these new cutting edge disability assistance technologies are often located in the regional hubs. Do your research and, if they are near your smaller company, go and meet with them face to face. What are they doing that you are not? What lessons can you learn from them and other companies? Connect, see theatre, see other companies, read about them and see their work. Go see assistive technology companies as well. What better PR for their stand-up wheelchair than for you to let one of your lead actors (who is in a wheelchair already, *not* a non-disabled actor) use it onstage for the season? Then track the audience reaction, get the feedback, what works? When you know what works for your company, then you are on the path to sustaining it.

We are all compelled to create a larger platform for the disabled artist in the arts community as well as to have discourse about how disability issues intersect with gender issues and transphobia and homophobia, racism, ageism and ableism. The sheer misunderstanding of the realities and abilities of all these marginalized groups, as well as the true benefits to be gained in working with them, has to start to be addressed on a systemic, academic level as well as a nationwide social, training, recruitment and employment level. We cannot bemoan the lack of talented actors, designers and directors with disabilities if we are not also in the serious business of committing to training, developing and employing them.

When I look at national organizations in the US such as the wonderful National Arts and Disability Council out of UCLA I am glad they are doing what they are doing, *but* often they themselves have to cancel or postpone their own training or advocation seminars because the group of teachers, advocates, speakers and trainers they use is small and they are often overwhelmed with the sheer volume of work. Granted, a young cadre of advocates and activists is out there in the US and is very active, but even they aren't getting enough encouragement, training and mentoring from some of the funders, universities, older advocates, writers and activists.

Perhaps then the greatest difficulty the disabled arts community has to battle is their own sheer diversity. There are so many different disabilities and so many sub-groups of activists that it often is hard to get them all to agree on something, or even a set vocabulary for that something. Oftentimes it is even difficult to get them all to agree on what a disability is and, with the acknowledgment that mental and developmental disorders are disabilities, this discourse grows even more broadly. Even within the disability community there is ongoing systemic, vocabulary and structural change about what defines a disability, what language we use and what the priorities are for activism and advocacy, education and outreach.

Every disabled group and subset of that group wants a piece of the performing and funding pie. I certainly understand that and agree we all should have it, but I also sometimes wonder if it might not be better to band together and fight for half the pie and then divide it up later? Twenty percent of the population is a huge community and the more the mobility impaired and deaf, the folks with CP and MS and those who are blind, the wheelchair users and those with autism, those with developmental and hidden disabilities and those who support and advocate for and with them can band together, the more we can all become a cohesive powerful group, one voice with the same priorities, the more we can begin to toss our 'twenty percent of the population' weight around as a much more solid political and social agent for systemic, academic, artistic, employment and creative change.

What about the ability to use creative change to sustain a theatre longer term when working with disabled artists only, as opposed to mixing both disabled and non-disabled artists? I continue to reply that in every single case when working with disabled artists I have seen it only maintain or increase box office revenue (meaning that if it is good theatre and not 'hey we are spunky and handi-capable!' audiences will come to see it). Were that not the case for my company, and if our box office revenue had plummeted, I still would have produced what we did anyway and waited for the world to catch up to us. My belief was and is that strong in regard to fully inclusive theatre.

There are also federal monies out there for inclusive theatre issues, accessibility, playwright development, closed captioning programs, etc. If you are ready to work with artists with disabilities, the money and the audiences are out there.

In this extreme digital age I often also get flummoxed at those who also claim that no grants can be found to apply for. Where are you looking? You have the greatest resource tool known, the internet, at your disposal and using it wisely can help get you the funding you need. Search under keywords, by disability, by accessibility, by time frame, by genre of production, by program or project idea, by city, state or region, by budget size, by your company size, by union contract, by subject matter. Audiences bring money in the door, but it is up to you and your development director to get the funders for the more substantial amounts (and for the status that state, private or federal funding can bring) and longer-term funding or endowments. Build upon your city and small grants wisely and in three years you will be getting state grants and three years after that, federal grants.

With community, federal, private, local, city, county and state funds there are nearly 140,000 grantmakers (check the Foundation Directory Online) across the USA. This does not include individual donors in your community who are not connected to a grant-giving group. Grants can be used to spearhead larger projects, as seed money for new projects, to increase access and recruiting, to pay new staff members, institute new training projects and so much more. If you do not have anyone on staff with a background in development and fundraising, then you must try to find someone, as applying for grants is an art unto itself and needs to be done correctly. The sky is indeed the limit, but you have to get started in researching, planning and applying for the funds.

Case Study 14: TBI and Cognitive Disabilities,
Nicu's Spoon Theatre, New York City

History

As do many theatres that work with inclusion or disability theatre, we taught and still teach classes in acting, auditioning, scene study, monologue work and more. At the end of each of the terms of classes we would usually have a showcase night with an invited audience of friends, casting people and company members. As we began the classes each year the usual end result involved showing memorized scenes or monologues – however, often students would not have the memorization capacity. A prime example was an actor I knew with two separate TBIs.

Plan

One actor in particular, let us call him Jim, had had not one, but two TBIs about four years apart and was left discovering that he had to redefine himself as a man and as an artist. It came as a surprise to him that he had no memorization capacity any longer. He would look at the words, know them, look up away from the page and they would be gone. This was emotionally devastating and physically taxing. He was an innately talented artist, really a good actor who had had a promising career at one time, an actor able to access his emotions very realistically (finding a male actor who can actually cry on cue is a rarity), and we looked for a way to solve this problem in order for him to perform for the showcase and feel good about his work. What could we do to help him?

See Chapter 16 for further details of this case study.

Chapter Action: Assess Your Theatre for Sustainability

Do a practical assessment yourself of your own theatre. How prepared is your theatre or theatre company to expand and become more inclusive? Access means not only being able to get on the stage and rehearse and perform, but also to attend as an audience member. In addition, true access means mental access to creation, access to decision making, new ideas, speaking out, doing a job, making decisions, having an artistic opinion. How well prepared is your group and membership to embark upon and embrace new ideas, new artists, new writers, new board members and new designers? On the technical side of things are the bars and/or restaurants that serve you and your patrons accessible around where you perform? (Or if your company goes to a bar after meetings, is it accessible for new members? If not, find a new watering hole.) If you have a bookstore or a theatre gift shop, can everyone access it? Equally important, can everyone exit it in an emergency?

Make a basic work list of things you would like to do and a basic wish list of things you dream about, what would you do if you could and what artists would you invite in? During (in some extreme cases) and certainly after each of our productions a full 'debrief' of the entire production process has always been held with the entire production staff, in person if possible and by email if not, to evaluate production values, the director, the actors, press and marketing, any internal issues, money and box office. This dissection and discussion enables us to remember lessons learned, not to make the same mistakes repeatedly, set higher goals and standards, issue invitations to new company members and to plot out a greater variety of productions in our future seasons (as it is only by understanding what you are doing that you can do something different). Do the same with your last production. Dissect it and learn from it. What can you learn? How can you use both inclusive/exclusive forms of public art as well as your performance art to shake things up?

Write down your fears about becoming accessible and inclusive if you need to and in the light of day, I guarantee you your fears are not as bad as you first thought, nor are there as many worries as you thought. Now start to dream big. Imagine you have all the money you need and artists of every kind to invite into your world. What can you do with that? What do you want to do? What productions or programming comes to mind? A theatre company assessment sheet and some examples of ideas and the types projects you can dream big with are on the companion website.

15

AFTERWORD

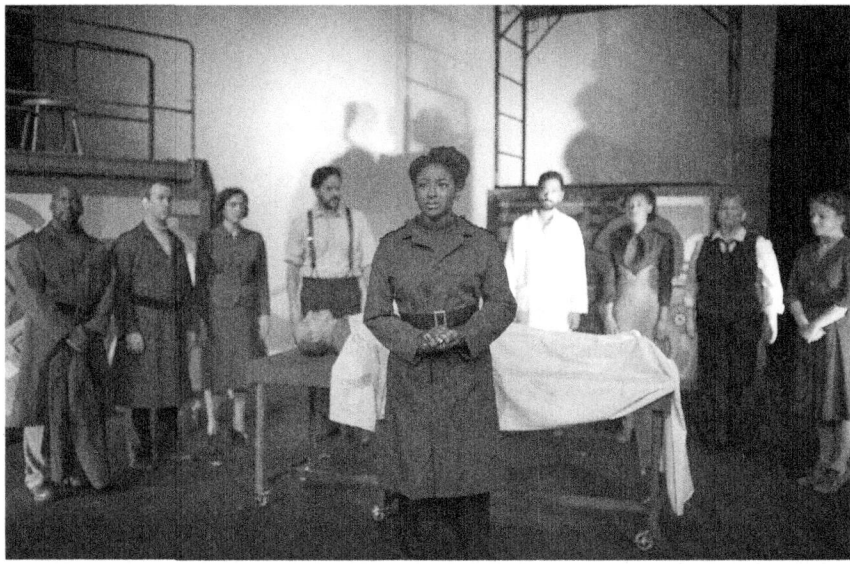

Figure 15.1 Universal Robots by Mac Rogers, 2016. L to R Tarantino Smith, Greg
Oliver Bodene, Tandy Cronyn, Jorge Cordova, Nikki Andrews-Ojo,
Neimah Djourabchi, Brittany N. Williams, Sara Thigpen, Hanna Cheek
and Jason Howard is lying on the table. (Photograph courtesy of Gideon
Productions.)

Turning poison into medicine is the spirit of the hero that
perseveres...whether it be Stephanie who is carrying on the life
and legacy of Nicu in believing in all of us, Sammy showing the
world a different way of seeing, Tony bringing humor to the
'bionic leg', or Rachel gracefully embracing a newfound fate.

Margaret Baker, actress, 2015, *Two and Twenty Troubles*
documentary

At the core, none of us were meant to be common.
We were born to be comets,
Darting across space and time —
Leaving our mark as we crash into everything.
A crater is a reminder that something amazing happened here —
An indelible impact that shook up the world.
                Donovan Livingston, Harvard Graduation speech, 2016

In October 2016, in an effort to increase media inclusivity and representation for disabled people, Towson University journalism professor Beth Haller (another great resource in the disability art world) and two associates co-founded the Global Alliance for Disability in Media and Entertainment. "People with disabilities should be telling their own stories," Haller said. "There should be actors with disabilities, directors with disabilities, journalists with disabilities." According to Haller (and she is right) the portrayal of people with disabilities by able-bodied actors is what the disability community calls 'cripping up.' In mid 2016 the Alliance of Resident Theatres/New York (ART/NY) began roundtable discussions and work groups for artistic and performance groups working with artists with disabilities; in that year, with the watchwords being 'diversity' and 'disability,' the artistic groups were multiplying in New York and were finally beginning to get some support.

However, in mid 2016 in New York City I watched as an audition monitor at an AEA union audition bent down and addressed an actress in a wheelchair in a saccharine baby voice, "Well, hi...how can I help you today? Do you want to audition for us?" and then stood back up perkily and addressed the person who had come in with the artist (who was not in a wheelchair) in a perfectly normal speaking voice. We have seen an active debate in 2016 of the perceived treatment or non-treatment of people with disabilities within the presidential race itself and what is very telling is that it sadly seemed to have no impact on the actual election. In Waterloo, Canada (granted, not the US, but still) a new musical 'Marathon of Hope' based on the life of Terry Fox, cast a non-disabled actor in the lead role when the entire point of the musical is his running a marathon as an amputee. An attached 'prosthesis' sits atop the actor's real leg (which is clothed in a black legging to make it 'disappear,' but in reality it only gives him the appearance of a tripod). One step forward and a half step back...

The above is all true. The Global Alliance is only one of many groups who will be watchdogging the issues and getting involved in casting in the years to come. Added to this is the fact that any inclusion on television or on stage is now heavily scrutinized to see if it promotes and supports inclusion in real life. Does the increased visibility of our veterans in such shows as 'Dancing With The Stars' and the like support them and show their reality? It certainly increases their visibility and makes people see and think and that, in my opinion, is never wasted energy. Their increasing visibility and how this vibrant populace is dealt with in the USA will be heavily scrutinized in the years to come.

However, the longer my company and other inclusive companies work, it seems there is more to be done and more areas and arenas in which to do it. I began the company in 2001 after realizing the enormous disparity between what many theatre companies, funders and artists said and what they actually did. However, after seventeen seasons I knew that a substantial mechanism for change is not only performance, but the exchange and revealing of information. Thus this book. I had to change my life, location and the company schedule to be able to write this book because the work is still out there and would demand my time if I did not. However, more new companies are emerging in New York and across the US and they are working with more and more marginalized groups and more artists with disabilities. My company continues to mentor a handful of younger, newer companies and often provides casting assistance across the US for television, film and for stage. We mentor actors, models, stage managers, designers, composers and playwrights.

Our 2017 season looks to move into an even more global arena with a long-term planning project, a multi-country live written and streamed project, GLOBE. Nothing like GLOBE has ever been done before and we are not even sure if it will come to fruition, however, it is the trying that matters. It is only because of the previous sixteen years of work and the benefits we have reaped that we can try to move into far more ambitious work. My company was created to take risks. We take risks and if we fail we are the richer for having taken the risks. If we do not fail then we never learn and never create art which can cause change. Your company can do the same and by the very nature of what theatre is, your company should be creating change.

What does this inclusive theatre work *really* offer to you, your company, your production, your actors and crew and the audience? What does this work really create within the drama school at your university? What are the outcomes you can expect if you use the best practices contained in this book in creating theatre? What we do is not therapy where we sit in a circle and talk about how we had hard times because of disability or color or age. We do not hold hands and sing hymns either. We work. We work like professionals and we make art. We speak to each other clearly and see each other for who we are. The vision of the project is paramount and all of us are, or become in the process, professionals joined by a common goal.

If it is, perhaps, in the end a little bit of therapy, then it is therapy of an indirect nature where it becomes about something bigger than the disability or inclusion, bigger than the artist or color or age, it becomes a larger project which we all work towards equally as collaborators. It becomes about the work and the play (as it should be) and the project and the group message. A by-product of this work is that it also serves to bolster further neuroplasticity and brain growth activity in artists of all kinds, those who are disabled and those who are non-disabled. Neuroplasticity and brain growth means change. Change. This work serves to be of a much greater motivator for everyone, makes for greater artistic investment and has a more lasting benefit for all of us than sitting and talking about, "How does being disabled (or black or gay) make you feel?" This work creates change.

It is not always perfect, it is not always warm and fuzzy. I recall one actress I worked with who was deaf who did a wonderful play reading with me (by Raymond Luczak) who always seemed angry at me and slightly suspicious of me for producing it, as I was not deaf. I was not sharing Deaf 'culture' with her, my whole theatre group was not fully deaf and she was a bit affronted by that, being angry as I was not deaf like her. She just could not put her finger on what my investment in this community was and what I was getting out of it as it was not my culture. Was it money? Notoriety? Neither, and thus she was baffled and a bit standoffish. We still produced the play with both hearing and deaf artists and she and the piece were wonderful, but I realized then that we collectively must continue to enable the co-ownership of inclusive art no matter what the disability, gender, race, age or lack thereof. Distractions like anger or a distancing (through word and action as well as thought) of those who do not share a membership in the same marginalized group as you will not only dull the creation of art, but the growth of spirit.

I have always wanted our productions to be the ones that do change the spirit, change the brain activity, change kinetic physicalities, change the artist and audience, change society, change the soul. I have wanted our productions to be the ones that the artists, designers and audiences remember years after they have seen them. Many actors or designers do show after show, year after year, so many in fact that it becomes a blur over the years. You ask them what their favorites are and their eyes glaze over because they cannot remember any of them. I want our shows to stand out from that blur for all the artists and designers, not just the disabled ones, because they were cast in a great role, because they learned about another artist's disability, because although they have one disability they played a character with a different disability entirely. Or because they learned something about themselves or their relationship to the world and their art. Or because their brain or body underwent a change and now they have something new they can do and carry with them or teach and share with other artists. Our shows must matter to both artists and audiences. It is not enough for us or you to simply do OK theatre. Box office revenue is not enough.

All of this is what you too can do, what your theatre group can do if you invest your time, sweat, blood, tears, sacrifice family time and make a commitment. You will make theatre that matters. Your shows, your university, your local or regional theatre must make this matter too. It is not enough to do 'Meh' theatre. Theatre has always been meant to be more than simple entertainment.

For those among you who are new directors with disabilities, do not let this hinder you in any way. Unless some aspect of the work is affected by your disability, it does not matter (and if it is affected, it can be altered or adjusted with very small effort). You must proceed in the assumption that you can have access anywhere. Again, assume access. Assuming access is a powerful thing. Send your résumé in and apply

for directing jobs and network, it is up to them to make the stage and
so forth accessible if you need it. If you are a designer, take the helm as
well and simply go for the jobs. It should not be an issue of 'disclosure'
anymore. You are artists and that is all you need to disclose, do not talk
yourself out of jobs before applying. Do not give up. Playwrights with
disabilities should submit like mad as well, but do not hold yourself
to only submitting to calls for playwrights with disabilities. Submit to
all the festivals. We must all start to '*assume and presume*' inclusion and
access. Nothing about us, without us. A tipping point will come. The
world then has no choice but to follow suit.

One of our company members, Phillip Chavira, went on to
become CEO of CastMe and a producer at Davelle, LLC, one of the
producers of *Eclipsed* on Broadway (with multiple Tony nominations)
and is a young champion of diversity in the industry. Both of his
ventures support multi-ethnic and experimental casting and he is
going on to carry one of the many torches for inclusive theatre.
How proud am I? This is one, only *one* of our company members
who carries this legacy into future work. The active choices we can
make now in regard to race and age and gender and disability can
illuminate plays and people and characters in new ways. These daily
choices can inspire writers, directors, company members, audience
members and young artists, board members and casting directors.
They can then inspire the future of this field. We know this from
experience. All it takes is the thinking of it and the doing of it.

A secret dream of mine (one of quite a few shows I would love
to direct) is to direct *Who's Afraid of Virginia Woolf?* but have it all co-
played with deaf and hearing actors and have Martha co-played and
signed by a large, scary black man. Yes, I realize a 'scary black man' is
a bad, racist and outdated stereotype (and something black men are
killed on our streets every day for being), but that is precisely why it
needs to be examined and put in front of an audience and precisely
why I would do it. Putting important issues in front of audiences
is what my company does. Perhaps I would have George then co-
played by a signing actor with a disability in a police uniform and
I would do this even if I was very certain it made folks think or get
angry, because then we have to examine what they are angry about.
We have to discuss societal, political and racial issues and embrace
possible change. In shaking things up we open 'set in stone' ideas,

societal problems, audience members' minds and we all see theatre and each other anew. The emerging artists this book addresses, and whom you should now hire and support, make theatre anew as well. They make us see and experience things anew.

The work you do as a company can empower and impact artists in ways that you and they may not even fully understand yet. In *Richard III* (2015) a lovely actress called Stephanie Gould played a few roles for me, including the Duchess of York and Norfolk. Stephanie has CP and has a weaker and shorter left side and arm. We hadn't talked about her CP and this arm, really, other than informationally and a little bit about how it impacted her childhood, but as we worked on the show I saw her own regimen of self-challenges, her mental drive to be better every day, to mentally and emotionally confront her own issues. There was a will of iron in her that people often do not see. As we began to work on Norfolk (whom she played with arm crutches) I opted to give her some moments of a bit of complicated and quick prop usage activity with her left hand and arm (which were already busy working with an arm crutch).

She worked like mad with this blocking and activity as I knew she would, and as she worked with it and mastered the prop and blocking work she became a bit emotional, so we sat down during a break to talk. I told her I knew it was frustrating. She began to cry and said that it wasn't that, it was that she really worked to not tax her left arm and usually nobody asked her to do tough things with it. I said, "I know, honey. However, you *can* do anything and everything with that left arm, just like with the right one. That is why I am asking you to do it, to challenge you." She began to cry again a little bit, and said "I know I can do it, but I didn't necessarily believe it until now." As of this writing she has even more deeply embraced her hard-work ethics and adapted her entire life (and lovely family video of herself and her parents) into a one-woman performance piece called *Walk With Me: A Surprisingly True Story* which successfully premiered in November 2016 in New York City. It is playing again in another run in 2017 and is one of the best solo shows I have ever seen. How many lives will she impact because of her work? How many minds will she directly change herself?

There is a depth of meaning inherent in working with artists with disabilities who have a bit more baggage than a 'bad day at the office.'

Living with a disability means that you have already girded your loins and faced fears most people have not faced. There is a richness of life experience, less bull and pomposity in general, and, if given a safe place to play and rehearse and make art, a creative belief in brand new artistic ways of being. Every time we embark on a new project idea or bring some new concept to a new production I find myself saying to the artists and staff involved, "OK, now just trust me, I know this sounds odd, but this is going to work." and god love them, they always do trust me (although I am sure they all must think I am out of my mind at times). Perhaps that is why they trust, because they have already dealt with so much and they are ready and willing to risk.

So, with a strong beginning base of mutual trust and respect the work then really does become a true springboard for new performance ideas and styles, meshes of performances for mixed groups (deaf, blind and hearing audiences simultaneously enjoying theatre for instance, all laughing at the same joke or crying at the same moment) and a well of boundless creation and discovery for both the artists and the audiences. We also build a platform for disabled artists to network and speak to each other about their lives, abilities, hardships and successes. Much of performance art concerns itself with the audience, and of course, we do too, but we also must concern ourselves with the artists first. If the artists are not secure enough to take a risk, then there is no true art for the audience to be changed by.

In our first production with co-playing in 2005, Mark Medoff's play *Stumps*, two of the actresses shared the role of Emily, a woman being abused and at one point in the play there was a large monologue about it. The normal choice would have been to have the speaking actress take the stage if there are two actresses. Instead, what I did was have the speaking actress sit behind the signing actress on a couch and wrap herself around 'herself' as she spoke the monologue with the signing actress in the forefront acting and being the stronger image. Granted, this subtle work with two artists playing one role asks more of an audience than just showing up. They must pay attention and think very hard about what they see and hear and feel and understand. They must re-examine their own preconceived notions about disability and about theatre and perhaps about themselves as human beings. This also asks of actors that they 'share' a role in a way they never have before and let egos fall away in that sharing, bringing with it beautiful and true shared acting choices.

The use of deaf actors, as well as blind actors or artists in wheelchairs, with CP or any disability, has to become thought of as the same as using any other non-disabled actor (small inroads are being made into this in 2016 in theatre and I would theorize some of the work with deaf actors stems from the Deaf culture being so strong and supportive, as well as the continuing amazing work from Deaf West Theatre in Los Angeles) and not just as interpreters or one-offs. Television is doing better in casting (kudos to *Speechless* on ABC) but still is light-years away from being truly inclusive. Hollywood, unfortunately (and I say unfortunately as Hollywood is the public face of American entertainment to the rest of the world) is a continuing vacuum of disappointment, casting and filming trite, badly written, 'poor disabled person' scenarios and then having nearly all disabled roles played by non-disabled actors. The current whitewashing of Hollywood and its color ignorant casting for major motion pictures is yet another indication of this insidious disappointment, as is the casting of non-LGBTQIA artists in gay or transgender roles.

Hollywood could and should be at the international forefront of this disability and inclusion movement and could substantially re-envision itself as a global leader in diversity, but Hollywood is horribly falling short. It takes the easy and box office sure (or so it thinks, look at the box office for *Me Before You*) steps in casting, not the new and bold choices. Until a unique and more energized generation of creators and casting people take over the helm in Hollywood, my prediction is that it will continue to fall short on this and many other diversity casting issues. (There are exceptions, however I am speaking of Hollywood as a whole.) A smart step forward would be to train within the LGBTQIA community and those from the disability community in apprenticeships in casting, but who will make the first step to do it? The challenge is here, pick it up.

Australia, on the other hand, has Kmart models with prosthetics and disabilities, and fashion models doing fashion shows with disabilities (Robyn Lambird and Madeline Stuart) and more advertisers working with disability (the recent National Disability Insurance Scheme commercial for instance). Great Britain had enormous advertising ads with disabled people for the 2016 Paralympics, many more than the USA. Many countries are doing much better than us in their casting and mainstreaming of actors, models, artists and ads and images of those with differing abilities. It is not all perfect, but they are trying, and most of the time that is where the US drops the ball.

My company has been compelled to open our brains and have a disabled artist take a lead role or be the main narrator for our new play reading series as we did for many years. Audrey Schading would show up with her service dogs (we worked with two of her dogs over the years) onstage and read with her braille reader and give her talents in being a part of something. How great it was. How audiences enjoyed it and her talent, with her beautiful voice and graceful presence (and those dogs, let's not lie). It benefited all of us.

For yourself, as a producer of artistic work, do not let *any* disability an artist has stop you from working with the artist. Mobility issues and the like you must work through with the artist to find the framework of what they can and cannot do or will and will not do. Just the same as with any artist. I have worked with many artists on the autism spectrum as well over the years and have delighted not only in their talent, but also in their ability to see the world differently and very often to articulate how they see it differently, or paint it differently, or write it differently. I adore the fact that these artists see the world differently to me and, for many of them, working with an inclusive company may be the very first time they encounter a place where someone really, truly is interested in how they perceive things as a creative being.

Many artists with disabilities, however, can also have their own ingrown societal misconceptions about other artists with disabilities, and that has been something we have been able to change just by having them work together. Often there may even be a disabled person who feels that certain other things are not 'real' disabilities. Someone with MS might not relate to someone with alopecia, serious dyslexia, stuttering or epilepsy as having a 'real' disability. One disabled artist might assume all wheelchair users have the exact same type of wheelchair or use their wheelchairs with the same amount of physical ease and mobility. Just because you are disabled doesn't mean you get the instant sainthood medal and immediately medically understand and fully relate to every other disability there is on the planet. Often non-disabled people do not understand this at all. "Oh you have MS? You must know John in LA, he has MS too!" "Um, no I don't know him. I live in Denver."

Creating a safe place that lets artists with differing physical, mental and neurological issues meet and work and change each other's perceptions by working together is a boon in any production situation, but even more so when working with a vast variety of disabilities and then finding ways they can combine and grow on an artistic platform. I really have overheard many wonderfully interesting conversations over the years about "Oh, your CP only affects your legs? Wow, mine does my legs and my speech, like I sound like I'm drunk sometimes!" or "Alopecia is what? Oh wow, you really do not even have eyelashes!" or "Yeah, well I was born without a leg so for me this is all I know, but man your thing is tough with losing it after having it." "I suffer from neurodiversity." "Neuro-what?" The sharing, the odd and sometimes dark humor ("What are you, blind?" "Yes, I am!"), it all draws us together and benefits the art and the artist and the human being.

Andrew Solomon, in his award-winning book *Far From the Tree*, tells us that in the US 'horizontal families' are growing in number. These are families of personal choice, not of blood. These are families of need and connection and shared abilities and understanding, not of money, genetics or power. Theatre companies are families that are inherently horizontal families and they must continue to become more diverse or we will suffer as a society. Often I have become sort of a parental figure to actors, as sometimes their parents have tried to minimize their disability or conform them to a preconceived notion of normal. While it is flattering, I do disabuse them of that pretty fast, as I am a taskmaster. I hug and love, but then it is back to work. I am not always a warm and fuzzy person. My concern for them is not as for children, but as fully formed artists. My concern now is for the world they enter, which must be ready to work with them.

The audience's benefits in your work are many as they get to see a rainbow of artists onstage and they do begin to understand that the world is made up of many types of people they may have not wanted to think about or had not taken the time to think about. Children's shows with a diverse cast not only teach children to appreciate different people, but to a disabled child who sees themselves reflected onstage it can be one of the most empowering moments in their young life. If you are a child with a disability and you see someone onstage with that disability, or even another disability, you see yourself differently. I have seen children blossom from happiness because, "The lady onstage has a crooked leg like me!"

As you introduce new plays into your company or onto your campus, why not introduce new artists in them? Or new playwrights? Introduce the training of new young directors, both disabled and/or knowing how to work with the disabled. Over our sixteen seasons we have probably given a dozen young directors the chance to work with a large disabled cast and staff and when they do move on to other work and companies the hope is that they will always retain that ability and open mindedness, the techniques and checklists, and will always have that be a part of their brain that might just say, "Hey, yeah I love that autistic actor, let's cast him in the lead role."

Over the years some of the artist's benefits after working with us have been that they have created their own companies. Gregg Mozgala has a small New York City company (The Apothetae) that actively encourages disabled playwrights and plays created about the disabled experience. Coupled with that is Gregg's own work as a writer, actor, teacher and speaker. Nick Linnehan has founded his own company (Identity Theater Company) which actively works with artists with disabilities and tours children's shows to schools. Phillip Chavira runs a company, Partly Cloudy People, that partners with a social cause and organization for each one of the plays they produce (like suicide issues), the play being about that specific cause.

In 2012 my company was also delighted to be one of the founding organizations of the Disability Cinema Coalition (DCC), based in Texas, which is a network of groups in theatre and cinema dedicated to the empowerment and inclusion of people with disabilities in the cinematic arts. Sammy, our company member, has crewed on their first coalition produced film, *Love Land*, and we continue to support them each year as they develop new projects.

We cannot forget the positive (and oftentimes very life-changing) impact that working with such diversity has on performers who are not diverse, not disabled. Many actors who are not disabled never look at a disabled person the same way after working with our company.

Many of the non-disabled artists who work with other companies then urge those companies to work with the disabled artists they have met during our shows (and many times they do). I choose and cast my non-disabled artists as carefully as I choose the artists who are disabled. Non-disabled actors who are high maintenance, easily prejudiced, closed-minded folks need not apply, and also do not last very long in our working process.

One of my favorite outcomes of this work is the 'intersectionality' of the diverse groups; how a person of color learns from someone in a wheelchair or a seventy-five-year-old writer learns from an LGBTQIA person. A five-year-old actress learns about CP or alopecia and never looks at 'different people' in the same way again. Every single one of these artists who learns from, or about, a disabled artist or designer is one more person who gets it, who will then welcome the chance to work with artists with disabilities again, or to cast them or go to see them in a show or to support the theatres which work with them. It truly is a snowball effect.

Another of the greatest benefits of all this work is one I never even realized at the time it happened, but only see now, and that is the impact it has had on my own child. This child grew up knowing blind people, people in wheelchairs, people with alopecia and CP and MS and who were deaf and so forth. Sam grew up with straight and gay and black and white and Hispanic and Asian people in his life. He never gave it a second thought that all his 'aunts' and 'uncles' were so very different. It has made for a kid who now, at fifteen years old, is a writer and artist and a champion for others and their rights as fellow artists and human beings. He also is a fervent animal rights supporter. He feels for and fights for the underdogs in the world and I could not be more proud of Sam.

As this book has an emphasis on our work with disabled artists, I have not given many examples of the rest of our rainbow of artists or work. However, our company diversity encompasses age, gender, race, nationality, sexual and gender identification and religion as well as disability. Disability is just one of the many ways in which we as a species fear we are all different, but in reality we are all more the same than we ever knew. There is a fellow human being inside each non-conforming body, inside each hue of skin color, inside each age and gender and religion. There are also some ways I haven't mentioned how we do certain things with a disabled artist because most of the time we do most of the 'certain things' exactly the same as with a non-disabled person. Many times you do not need to solve a problem at all, just relax and proceed as you would usually.

Do I have any last ideas? Always. About a million a day, actually. Arts festivals (and I address the non-disability arts festivals) across the US should actively make sure a percentage of their exhibitors and attendees are disabled (ten percent would be a good starting goal). National and local arts conferences should also actively recruit and invite disabled performers, speakers and teachers as well as merchandise sellers. A system of apprenticeships should be continually happening with the fine arts creators in the USA. Take a disabled apprentice to teach pottery and silk screening and woodworking. I bet a potter who is blind or deaf would make amazing art. Arts grants on every level from national to local should actively invite disabled applicants and make use of smart and relevant technology so that online applications are accessible to all. Elected officials should be investing their discretionary funds into education and the arts. All online forms should be fully accessible. A blind applicant should be able to hear an online form ask questions and type in their replies in real time.

A national database of all artists with disabilities, union and non-union, both in the fine and performing arts could also be created so that they can all be sought out, supported and recruited and cast and collaborated with. Celebrities need to be giving their money to groups to do all of this instead of purchasing new houses. Universities need to be putting these issues and ideas on their development schedule. Politicians need to have arts programming on their docket. Most groups working in the field of inclusive theatre are like my company, a 501c3 nonprofit, so it is all tax deductible. We can all make this happen. What ideas do you and your group have? Think outside the box, think ahead of the technology, think beyond the status quo.

One last story. Kate Breen and Thea McCartan, two terrifically talented actresses, were co-cast in *Stumps* in the role of Emily and had worked very well together in rehearsals. As we were starting to see with the rest of the pairs of co-players, an instinctive emotional telepathy was happening onstage where at times they didn't have to watch each other for cues, they just knew when to do something (even if it was a new acting or movement moment it seemed it would happen to both artists at once). However, in rehearsals we had interpreters to help out with day-to-day communication if needed.

One day these two actresses told me that they planned to meet outside the rehearsals to go over the part and discuss some moments together. I was a bit concerned because the speaking actress (Thea) only knew a handful of signs at that time, so I asked them if they needed a facilitator to go and meet with them to interpret for them as they worked on the role. The two young women looked at each other and about a million unspoken thoughts zinged between them at once. "No," Thea said. "We'll figure it out. We understand each other just fine." I was so happy to hear that. I just thought, *that's* what doing this work is all about.

Case Study 15: Gideon Productions, New York City

Sean Williams Executive Producer and Co-Founder

Author's note: This is the only case study in this book written from the perspective of a theatrical production company that does not normally work with or for disabled artists. This is a company that is trying and finding their way and is very honest about their efforts. For that, and their creativity and the path they are on to work with and for disabled artists, I applaud them heartily. They are doing what I urge all companies to do in this book, they are taking the first steps.

The mission statement for Gideon Productions is a paragraph long but there is one sentence in the middle that we use as a crucible for any piece we're considering producing – "We explore what's strange about being human and what's human about being strange." To this end, we've told stories time and again about people who, for one reason or another, aren't moving through the world the same way everyone else is.

But we'd never taken the next logical step – to reach out to the communities who literally experience the world in a different way and who haven't been targeted by us as audience members. So we started brainstorming. A performance for the deaf? Of course! There was already a roadmap for that. Can we do a performance for the blind? I bet we can. What about people who can't normally come to the theatre, people with Tourette's syndrome or social anxiety disorders, can we reach them? And what about the group I belong to – those who can't see theatre because their kids can't be left alone and babysitting is expensive? We decided to try to reach all four of these communities.

My first and best phone call was to Marielle Duke at Adaptive Arts Theater Company in New York. Her organization is working to bridge the gap between disability and the arts. She helped to spearhead nearly every single aspect of these outreach programs for us.

Performance for the Deaf

Obviously, in New York there is already a roadmap in place for this, and I'm also lucky that one of my oldest friends is an interpreter. We contacted Dylan Geil and Lusanne Massaro and only once they enthusiastically agreed to do it did we realize we'd stumbled on to two of the best interpreters in New York. Before the interpreted performance, they sat in the back of the house for two other performances and practiced switching parts back and forth. To reach the deaf audience, we contacted New York Deaf Theatre

(NYDT), Theater Breaking Through Barriers, Hands On and several other organizations. We even donated tickets to a fundraiser for NYDT in order to help them while they were spreading the word.

Performance for the Blind

After some research, we found an organization called Sound Associates that has hardware and software to provide what is called 'D-Scriptive' service. Through this, a blind person can wear a single ear bud and they can listen to a narration that accompanies the performance. The narration can either be recorded or performed live. To reach the blind audience, we contacted the American Foundation for the Blind and followed up with Theater Breaking Through Barriers (who for many years worked exclusively with blind artists). We also found a lot of support from the people who work at the Theatre Development Fund in New York, even though they generally only give official support to organizations that are working with them in a professional capacity. These programs inspired a lot of people to want to help.

Audiences with Invisible Disabilities

One of our initial goals was to create accessible performance specifically targeted to audience members who struggle with social interactions. We planned to create a 'Social story' on the website – a clear, step-by-step guide for patrons new to Gideon Productions or for whom this would be their first theatre experience.

We talked about creating special seating for any patrons who may need a break during the performance and spoke to the theatre about where this break could occur. We began the conversation about how to prepare our actors and designers for a performance with audience members who may not relate to the theatre in the same way we are used to (or we have learned to expect). Our hope was to create a fully comfortable experience for individuals who traditionally experience difficulty entering new spaces, particularly spaces bustling with people. For people who wanted to experience theatre but didn't feel a physical theatre space was a safe space for them, we began talking to AEA about doing a livestream performance.

Parents with Small Kids

This was, in a lot of ways, the easiest because I knew if I couldn't find any other solution, I had about fifteen people who could sit with the kids during the performance. Right away, The Sheen Center (where our show was being produced) offered us the use of several rooms on site. This allowed us to split up the kids into two groups: ages 4–8 and ages 8–12. The production was recommended for kids thirteen and up, so older kids could just watch the show with their folks.

Facebook and personal email was the best way for us to reach parents. There are many, many groups on social media that will pass along offers to parents and we have a huge network of theatre parents that we're close with. So many organizations are out there with teaching assistants who are trained to take kids through projects and programs and we had an outpouring of help from places like the New Victory Theater, the Lincoln Center and New York University.

So, we found ourselves a few weeks before opening with everything set in place. We had a dedicated performance for the deaf, a performance for the blind, a performance for parents with small kids and an educated, articulate approach to audiences with invisible disabilities. Our next step was implementing the ideas and organizing the audiences for the performances.

See Chapter 16 for further details of this case study.

16

CASE STUDY OUTCOMES

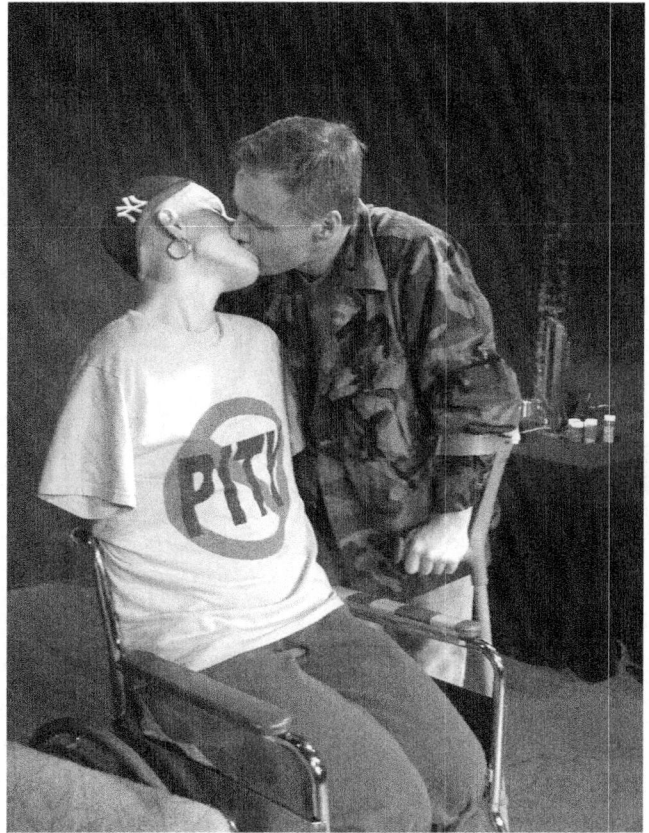

Figure 16.1 Kite Cut Loose in the Middle of the Sky, by David Greenberg, 2008. Margaret Baker and Mark Armstrong. (Photograph courtesy of Nicu's Spoon Theater Company.)

These case study outcomes are as varied and wonderful as the groups that provided them. In almost all of the cases the immediate and long-term outcomes were good. However, in some cases they were not and those cases are as important, if not more so, than the successful ones. The important take-away from all the cases is the trying, the risking, the creating. Even when we fail we create change.

Case Study 1: A Seizure Onstage

What do you do? How do you save your company, save the show, save the actor and still keep your profits?

So, the actor, let's call him Bob, began having a grand mal seizure, everyone froze and luckily that night my mother (who is a medical person) was in the audience. She looked at me, I nodded, and she jumped onto the stage just as the actor playing Atticus ran out onstage and put his credit card between Bob's teeth. I also looked into the booth at my stage manager and she already had the telephone moving toward her mouth. My lighting designer was on the phone as well. They were all very prepared, considering this was our second show as a company. I then stepped in front of the audience and said, "Folks, I would like to ask you to step out into the lobby for about ten minutes and have a glass of wine, our treat, as we deal with this moment. I will keep you in the loop!"

All the audience members got up and went to the lobby where our staff (quickly briefed by me) began to pour wine and offer reassurances. Our stage manager let me know EMTs were coming, then I went to the cast and explained what was up and that we would see what the EMTs said and then see where we were. The EMTs were there very fast and my mom gave them all the information along with Bob, who was post-seizure but exhausted. After a check-up they recommended we send him home as he needed to sleep. While we did some great audience misdirection and I spoke to them, the stage manager got Bob out the back door and in a cab to go home. I told the audience that we were canceling the night's show, we apologized, but this was a risk we gladly took in order to work with the artists we did. I invited them to have another glass of wine while I spoke to the other actors and we made out rain checks for the audience members to all come back and see it another night. They were told they would be given priority seating if they redeemed the rain checks.

I then told the cast, as the audience left, to go home. They took it harder, but since they loved Bob, they understood as best they could and went home. We issued forty-five rain checks for two tickets each that night and every single one was redeemed during our run. Every single audience member came back and saw the show. That's a pretty great audience. This one night was the only performance in seventeen seasons, forty mainstage shows and forty-five reading workshops that we have ever canceled.

Granted we were lucky my mother was there and had medical training, but my staff had common sense and we had been well prepared by our work. Another element that I feel is vital to how smoothly we made it through this crisis is that every one of my staff knew I trusted them and knew they were prepared so there was very little, "Oh, I better check with Stephanie before I take any initiative" happening. They knew what to do and they did it like professionals. The actors also responded accordingly. However, there are a number of ways this could have been an absolute mess and we could have alienated the audience as a whole. Instead, many of them became funders and long-term supporters after this show. The audience felt included as well, a part of the moment and the situation and not on the outside. I talked to them at all times and they appreciated the honesty. Inclusion also means including your audiences.

Case Study 2: Stage Manager in a Wheelchair

How could we get Marco up there? Did his chair have to go up there too? How did we solve it?

There are two solutions for this one. The first we had used, not with Marco, but years earlier with a tech person in a wheelchair. It was an exceptional solution, not because of it being complicated, but because of the tech person and their physical fitness and their manual chair. This was a tech person who was in and out of his chair all the time and very fit in his upper body, but could not get up into the booth. So we built what I called a 'sled.'

The sled was basically like a real sled except that it slid (was pulled from above actually) up the steep stairs into the booth area, the person was unstrapped from it and it was tucked away while he went to work. We could do this only because he had no spinal problems and was very fit and was used to the physicality of being out of his wheelchair.

Solution number two was what we did with Marco. Marco had an electric wheelchair and as mentioned before these are heavy monsters! He also pretty much needed to work from it, as most electric wheelchair users do. No worry. We re-routed the entire bit of electrical and wiring and connections we needed to run all of the multimedia for the show and we created the multimedia space offstage by the dressing rooms. Marco had a line of sight onto the stage and ran the multimedia from there for the entire performance run.

Many companies would not have bothered to do all that rewiring (or possibly would not have hired Marco to begin with) as it was time consuming, but I made sure we did it because that is what we do and it was important for Marco and his future career that he know how to run things like this. He needed the experience. He has since moved on to being an ASM for *Hamlet* in New York City with other actors who have worked with us and he is stage manager for the upcoming New York City Disability Pride. For him, as a disabled stage manager, it becomes about connections and recommendations, what he has already done and *what he can do*. He can now run multimedia for an enormous show, because we made sure he could.

However, in Marco's future stage management career this is something he must take into account every single time he accepts a job. Where is the rehearsal?

Where is the show? Is it wheelchair accessible? Is there a ramp? He can organize, coordinate and delegate, but he cannot assist with set building or running around much. He cannot build his own ramp. Unfortunately most of the time, even in New York City, there is no access and no ramp and one has to be built or he has to turn the work down. This is not his fault, it is ours, it is the architects and theatre owners. How can he build a career if once he is hired he cannot get into the spaces?

Case Study 3: Disabled Artist as Villain

How can we make the show go on, with Henry, with no ticket losses, with something inventive that we could do quickly that did not require recasting or re-blocking the entire show?

Well, my choice was this: I broke the role of Richard into two parts and we promptly had auditions for another actor. I was looking for an anti-Richard, tall and with a voice to die for. We found it in a young actor named Andrew Hutchinson. We worked him into the show and I took over directing for this last week and then we went into production.

This review from www.shakespeareteacher.com in 2007 explains it all for you.

> I had the pleasure of seeing *Richard III* at Nicu's Spoon Theatre. I had a wonderful experience, and I would recommend it to any fan of the play (it's my favorite) who is in the New York City area.

The title role was played by Henry Holden, who ... used crutches to get around the stage. This was presented as Richard's deformity. However, the actor skillfully embodied such a deformity of spirit in the role that the artificial leg was quickly overshadowed. This physicality was especially important, since Holden only spoke the lines that Richard speaks to the audience. When Richard was in public, his lines were spoken by a second actor, Andrew Hutcheson, who was positioned upstage left with a lectern and a reading light, while Holden remained as the physical Richard.

Typically, such production concepts turn me off immediately, but it worked particularly well here, in no small part due to the richly resonant voice of Hutcheson who overflowed the small house with Shakespeare the way it was meant to be performed. ... Also, having two actors playing Richard highlighted the contrast between Public Richard and Private Richard. The director ... also had the freedom to underscored the more poignant moments by having a character deliver a line addressed to Richard to Hutcheson instead of Holden, or to have both actors speak a line in unison. And Hutcheson turning off his reading lamp to signify Richard's death was a nice touch.

So, there you have it. Much easier said than done, to be sure, but it was an exceptional experience for us all and we got to work with two wonderful actors. Henry would eventually move back to LA, but Andrew did many more shows with us and went to our off-Broadway contract with us in 2008.

Case Study 4: Dionysus Theatre, Houston, Texas

So, we at Dionysus Theatre, after a month of arduous searching for a young, African-American girl who was either blind or sight impaired ended up finding our young actress in the unlikeliest of places. Not in the disabled community or schools where we had been searching, but in a mainstreamed class in a non-disabled school. The principal of the school heard about it from a friend of a friend and recommended the girl who got cast. Not only was she cast, but she was also mentored by the older actress and her confidence rose and so did her grades. *but* the take-away in this case is the community and Dionysus's reputation. Dionysus did not find this actress through their traditional ways of searching, this actress was found and recommended solely on the strength of the theatre's long-time good reputation.

Case Study 5: Can an Actor Who Is Deaf Speak?

What is your step-by-step checklist to getting Dax to performance?

1 Vocal work – humming and making mouth movements, reading lines silently but moving the lips. This was private work outside rehearsal with Dax and I.
2 Having the cast memorizing his lines and theirs for the scenes. This was in preparation for later scenes where an actor might repeat something Dax said.

3 Vocalization and enunciation early and making sure seventy percent of the vocalization exercising was done with full cast doing it as an exercise (thus it was a group effort with group support).

4 Private breathing and sound work as well as emotional support. Even if you do not speak habitually you still do make sound (deaf artists are frequently the noisiest people I know!) and use breath, so we worked with ways to capitalize on what sounds he already did make without thinking about it.

5 Carefully choreographed signals for Dax for all entry and any other cues so that Dax owned his full performance, was confident about it, was in control and was not reliant on being cued by anyone at any time.

6 Giving Dax specific things to do with his hands onstage, which the text helped with a lot in specifying prop use, so that he would not have them subconsciously sign as he acted.

7 We did extensive text work with the full cast on the subtext of him being born deaf in the play and never being taught to sign and in what ways did that manifest itself in how the family treated him? (Did one family member echo Dax's speech? Did another ignore him entirely? Did one pick on him?) How did we use the lines in the play to bolster our theory?

8 Working in specific moments of pantomime (not signing) about only very specific things vital to the text that we felt Dax might mime as the deaf character in moments of high emotion.

9 Careful press information releases (*The New York Times* did a marvelous interview with Dax and the cast and reviews were great) and very careful discussion with Dax about his thoughts and ideas on PR in the Deaf community.

10 Constant support, open discussion and a tight community of support both in and outside rehearsal. Dax carried expectations from the Deaf community with him and we were all aware of that and fiercely protective of him, as was his wonderful family.

Case Study 6: Snow White *and* Richard III

Did I ask her to do it and if so, how? Or did I opt to let it go?

Time and time again I really feel lucky on things like this as I had known Rachel for four years before I had this situation come up. She knows me as someone who is honest and upfront about everything and someone who is deeply invested in her as an artist. So, we had a talk. I told her my overall thoughts for the battle and that I really wanted every single actor in the battle as I had really wanted to push the actors and audience into a new place of seeing what all bodies can do and how powerful disabled bodies and minds can be.

I then talked about her as an artist and her strength and her story and said, "I have an idea for you in the battle, but it may not be right, or you may not be comfortable with it. You *know* I will not do anything that makes you uncomfortable so can I tell you the idea and then you can punch me if you hate it?" We laughed and she said of course I could tell her. So, I did.

She listened thoughtfully and then thought for a moment (of course, I had no idea then what she was thinking) and then her face broke into a smile like the sunshine and she said, "*Oh my god! I love that*! I get to beat him to death? Awesome!" To this day when people who saw the play talk about the battle scene someone *always* says, "Oh, I loved when the gal who played Anne took her leg off and beat that little dude to death. That was amazing!"

Be honest, always start from honesty, make the artists safe and ask them what you need to. In the rare times they say no, have a secondary idea about the same moment, or ask them for an idea, and keep working and talking until you find something that works for them and you.

Case Study 7: Think Outside the Box for Accessible Sets and Non-Standard Staging

What could we do to turn it all more on its head and go against expectations?

As I said the movement patterns were very complex in staging this with ten actors, but we also had a wheelchair and there are certain things you must do so that a wheelchair can move, turn, etc. both on- and offstage. So, again turning things on their head I said, "Let's operate opposite the usual assumptions that will be made with the set because we have a wheelchair. Let's not worry about designing the set specifically for actor movement patterns as those are growing organically and can be put together onstage easily." (As this was our first co-played project we didn't know as much physically organic work would come out of this piece when we began.)

My choice then was to go against the common thought of the day and make sure the wheelchair had the run of the upper level, not the ground floor. The common theme of keep that wheelchair on the ground and solid was tossed aside (in the co-playing we had two actors playing the role of the wheelchair user and one was standing and was very physically strong and would 'spot' for the other in the chair). We let that wheelchair powered by two actors, one in it and one behind it, go all over the upper level of the set. This choice defied the norms and had a great side effect as well. In staging with actors in wheelchairs, you must always be aware of whether they can be seen by the audience. If they are on the audience height level then they are often blocked from view and you must alter blocking. This new crazy 'aloft' staging for a wheelchair user had the added benefit of the wheelchair user always being within audience sightlines. (This issue of an actor in a wheelchair, or an actor who is a little person, needing to be seen by an audience is one you must be fully aware of at all times. Sit in your own audience, can you see everyone?)

Case Study 8: Opening the Door

Design concepts at Phamaly Theatre Company

Central to the Tin Girl persona is the metal body that surrounds her. Mallory was able to seamlessly use the actor's wheelchair as the foundation for her tin costume. This made the wheelchair as theatrical as the costume itself, while also ensuring the costume wouldn't hinder the actor's movement. Not hiding it, not highlighting it, but using it as a central element in the design combined with the character's need to oil her axle informed the actor and the play in a new light.

Likewise, the actor playing the lion was able to purchase new glass eyes – of course designed to look like a cat's eyes – to embellish the rousing and impressive body suit he was wearing. Again, focus wasn't pulled directly to the actor's eyes, but the creativity of the design element combined with the rest of his outfit resulted in a truly incredible costume overall.

The key to solving the problem of accessibility in design is to embrace the obstacle, and work with the actor. Use the lack of physical access onstage purposefully, as a key metaphor for a character's economic background and inability to gain position; or use an actor's mobility device as a representation of freedom. This will allow the actor the opportunity to explore these metaphorical design elements physically.

Embracing the obstacle not only means applying a design concept to a character, but working with the individual to determine the best way to apply that concept – even if the inclusion elements in the design are meant to protect or be concealed.

Case Study 9: A Large Disabled and Diverse Cast in
Technical Rehearsal

So, how did we do it? Without mangling the cast?

If you are running special effects like fog or smoke or strobe lights, do everyone a favor and run these first many times with any stand-ins before the cast is there so this can be run once or twice at most with disabled (and older and younger) actors or artists and staff with asthma, sight or breathing issues. Do not run fog machines (or strobe lights which can bring on epileptic seizures) even five times or more with artists it can affect adversely.

We did all of our testing without the cast. We used those of our tech crew with good lungs and myself and volunteers and we set the lights and sound and ran the fog, and ran it and ran it. We decided how much we needed, so how long it should run. We set everything at approximate levels and then I stepped out and went into the audience to double check the look and had folks move around to all areas actors ended up in. Then we opted for a bit less time running it, knowing it would seem more dense with bodies in it. We ran all this a bit before folks even arrived and also ran the fast opening of the back and side doors for the clearing of the fog (both for the artists and audiences sake!).

Once actors arrived we ran the sequence twice with the full cast and then did not run it again until we ran it in the actual performance. There were a bit of notes and tweaking and we ran it one last time after the show and that was that. *Any* heavy tech should be run without actors if possible – use volunteer bodies or interns, but spare the actors wear and tear unless you really need to use them for something specific.

Case Study 10: Phamaly Theatre, Denver, Colorado

In the 2006 production of *Man of La Mancha*, Regan Linton (announced as the new Artistic Director of Phamaly in late 2016) portrayed the role of Aldonza, traditionally torn from her horse and left in a ditch. Instead of being ripped from a horse, she was ripped from her wheelchair; instead of being left in a 'ditch,' she was left onstage. Audiences had to be open to viewing the new and very real staging of this moment. Regan, too, in the role, had to be willing to allow the audience to view her vulnerably; and of course it would be irrational to assume that any actor would (or should) be willing to make such a statement, regardless of ability. But audiences were astounded to find Regan outside of her wheelchair – outside of the audience's perception of safety – and left alone to pull herself along the stage-floor to sing a powerful rendition of the famous song *Aldonza*.

Such a statement would not have been possible without the inclusion of safety elements within the scenic and costume designs to protect Regan's body; and working in close cooperation with the director, stage management and most important of all – Regan.

Overall, inclusion of actors with disabilities opens up an entirely new world of design possibilities for any production. Embracing the actor's talents – disabilities and all – can allow each artist to explore the material more deeply than ever before. The concepts that will blossom are easy to find. When the actor and designer work together, the accommodations needed for each concept are easy to capture. The design and concept potential is endless and exciting, but the hardest part – truly – is opening the door to the possibilities.

Case Study 11: A Blind Actor and Discovering Colors

So, what was the solution, the 'take-away' for this situation? This was, fortunately, one of the times when we had the time to ponder and think about this. So, being the director of the piece (and thus knowing I was going to impose my own notions of the play on the text anyway) I opted to meet the actor and grab a juice and head into Central Park. We sat and I told him, "I am going to try something and let's see if it makes you think colors." Knowing my inherent wackiness, he was game to try anything.

We spent about forty minutes in the park where I used his smell, touch, taste and hearing to give him my interpretation of colors. A sprig of grass with a small mint leaf in it for 'GREEN' ("Mmm, can I eat all this? Green is yummy."), a slow swipe of an ice cube across the back of his hand for BLUE. A nip on the end of a chili for RED. A bite of a sugar-dipped lemon for YELLOW. A recording of someone screeching on a saw instrument for STORM TOSSED BLACK AND GREY. A small hand bell ring for SILVER and so forth. We had a great time and watching his face as he processed each taste or feel or smell was an education for me as well.

We had no idea if it was just us having a great time in the park or if it would actually impact his monologue. However, when the next time came for him to do the monologue in rehearsal he stopped a few words in, paused, started to smile and then re-started the monologue going more slowly, addressing each color in a way that had us all in tears. The colors had not only become clear to him in a way that stuck with him and mattered to him, but had become clear in a way that they were re-made real again, seen and felt again, for us as audience members watching. This was also something he said he, "Could carry with me wherever I go now." As usual, with honest collaboration and exploration it is a win all around.

Case Study 12: That Uppity Theatre Company and the 'Think Tank' Project

I said to the audience, "Who doesn't like to go to a ball game?" And asked everyone including the audience to sing *Take Me Out to the Ballgame* with us. St Louis is a big baseball town so they connected with this idea right away. I then introduced the audience to our ball team and described the various elements that we might encounter at a ball game, including the peanut seller, and cued one man with frontal lobe dementia to be our peanut seller. "Peanuts, get your peanuts!"

We even had someone do the infamous wave with our theatre group as well as the audience. For a little feminist fun and to promote gender equality, I had one of our two women in the group be the person who hit a home run, while the social work interns coached her to run the bases. The audience loved it.

Then I talked about how everyone in the group was patriotic and had served their country in some way or been married to someone who did. And we all marched in place as a prequel to singing *God Bless America*, complete with gestures that again were coached.

The audience members sprang to their feet, applauding and cheering, many wiping away tears. I think they were overjoyed to see their loved ones enjoying themselves and they also understood that the performance was our gift to them, our way of saying thank you to partners, husbands and wives and children, siblings, neighbors and friends who help care for people with Alzheimer's and early stage dementia.

As the performance was our last official time with the group, I had asked them to designate a class valedictorian to make a little speech. They selected a former high school drama teacher who lost some of his words during his speech but none of his emotion or commitment. He cried talking about how much he loved the class and the performance and how it was proof that he could still act and that he felt very alive during our time together.

We had a little graduation ceremony and one by one, each person came up so they could be individually recognized and be given a rose. Backstage, which was just a little room where we had gathered in a community center, they were elated and not wanting to say goodbye to me or our social work students or to each other.

It's interesting that when the Alzheimer's Association first said they also wanted me to create a performance at the end for caregivers, they wanted multiple assurances that I would not make any of the participants look foolish. I was taken aback by the way they framed that request and I said, "Of course I won't make anyone look foolish. I never make anyone look foolish onstage and I don't make anyone do anything."

It was odd because they were the ones that had approached me, knowing of my reputation for working imaginatively and supportively with a variety of populations, including some whom had been traumatized.

I had no idea what would happen when I agreed to teach the class or to create a performance. I was open to all the possibilities. It was clear that our work together was therapeutic in a variety of ways and provided community and enhanced creative capacity. So not long after our performance, in my final debriefing with the program director who had hired me, I suggested we continue the project. She said there was no additional funding. I said I would either do it pro bono or find outside funding, that the group had asked me to continue. Then she said, they were grateful for my work, but that we had just been one module. They were doing visual arts next.

I tried to explore a few additional options but she wasn't open to them. It was heartbreaking and in that moment, I realized how our educational institutions and community programs fail so many, because they are often inflexible and either do not recognize or are threatened by innovation.

So many lessons learned through my work with Think Tank: how to expand contemporary definitions of performance; how to work effectively and pleasurably with this population; how deeply people benefit from this kind of work. And also, most notably, how a nonprofit can lack imagination or be operating out of fear and cut short real opportunities that could serve their constituencies with love and respect and skill.

Case Study 13: The Glass Menagerie

It had been a few years since I had worked on the role and knew I could approach it only from where I was now as an artist and a person. The more I prepared, the more I realized that I had been complicit in perpetuating every stereotype ever written about Laura. More importantly, I realized if I were fortunate enough to land the iconic role, I had a responsibility to myself to dig deep to find the ways in which we were similar rather than focusing on our differences, but more importantly, a responsibility to Laura (and to Tennessee Williams) to do her justice – to understand her, to honor her, to love her, free from any preconceived ideas and judgment. Once I understood that, my primary job would be to get out of the way and allow Laura to speak through me: my mind, my body, my heart, my soul. Just as I have for every role I play.

The audition was a dream. Thirty seconds in, I could literally feel the energy in the room shift. The director was focused, engaged. The reader was moved. The casting director knew she had made a mistake. After reading five plus pages of the 'Gentleman Caller' scene, I left the room. A moment later, the casting director, director and reader walked out of the room. The casting director said, "We were just discussing how wonderful you are." The director hugged me. I left, elated. An hour later, my agent called to say I had been called back. When I returned the next day, I learned they had called back only two women. The first was already in the room when I arrived and I heard a steady stream of laughter throughout her audition. I remember thinking, "If I don't get this part, I should probably stop acting."

Luckily, I didn't have to. I booked the job. When the casting director called my agent to make the offer, she asked, "Was that the actress you wanted me to see and I refused?" "Yes," he said. "I'm sorry," she said, "I was wrong."

From that moment on, I committed myself fully to Laura. We became less and less distinguishable from one another over the course of rehearsals. Her vulnerability, dreams, invisibility, generosity, isolation, beauty, imagination were mine. My joy, longing, physicality, empathy, pain, wisdom, fear, desire were hers. For sixteen performances, audiences watched Laura struggle to sit on a cushion and scoot across the floor. They watched her blossom in the presence of her singing pirate, fall on top of him as they waltzed and have to accept his help to get to her feet while searching frantically for Freckles, who had flown across the floor into the wings. When her heart soared with a single kiss, so did the audience's collective heart. When her heart shattered, their hearts shattered, too. The cast wept openly through every curtain call. So did the audience.

Case Study 14: TBI and Cognitive Disabilities

In the rehearsal process with Jim, watching him excel emotionally and embody every second of his work within both scenes and monologues we had given him to work on, we did struggle with how best to get him off book. Until we learned a lesson. I had an epiphany. There was no defining requirement for him or anyone to be off book and memorized, none at all. There was no need to adhere to any convention for us. An audience wants to see good acting, real emotions, living in the moment and that was what this inherently honest actor had. If we gave this performance to the audience they would accept it, follow it and enjoy it.

Ultimately we realized that to put any continued emphasis on memorization for him would neglect the enormous gifts he did have and would create such a stressful rehearsal and work process that it might indeed destroy his energy, the gifts he had and the remarkable progress he was making. Thus the rehearsals became about how and when to refer to the text, how and where to hold it, working on the real moments, blocking and concentrating on the acting, which is what it should be about anyway. The subsequent showcase and reception was wonderful and he ended up being the quiet, shy star of the night as his true talent shone through. Though he was later to leave acting for good and have many TBI-caused emotional and health issues, this remained an apex night for him and one he referred to often, even as his TBIs continued to impact his life and relationships.

Case Study 15: Gideon Productions, New York

Our production of *Universal Robots* was opening in June 2016 and by the beginning of May we were set to implement our community outreach initiatives. The interpreters were in place for our performance for deaf audiences, we had the devices on hold for blind audiences, our venue, The Sheen Center, had provided us with space for our Parents Initiative... It was all falling into place. So we sat down to prepare the Invisible Disability Outreach.

Again, Marielle Duke from Adaptive Arts was an enormous help. We started writing out the Social Story and planning for the alterations in the staging and audience interaction... But after a few weeks of work, it began to dawn on me that this was more than we could accomplish. The play was simply not designed to work with these modifications and when we looked at our production team we had to admit that we didn't have the manpower.

Our production company has been incredibly lucky in many ways. The press has consistently been kind to us and our audiences have been passionate and supportive. But this gives the illusion that we're a well-organized team with a solid infrastructure and we're just *not*. We're essentially just a few people who rely on the generosity of a lot of people.

This community-based approach to creating theatre works well only if we ask for things people are comfortable giving and if we can pay people back with opportunities they would enjoy. The people we work with have never done this kind of outreach, and didn't have the first clue how to help. After some soul-searching, Marielle and I canceled this initiative.

We still had three other programs to work on, so I first turned my focus reaching out to the Blind Community. I spent hours and hours on outreach, via email, texting and letter writing. And I was so frustrated that I wasn't hearing back. We had set up a special performance, we had invested time and money, why wasn't the Blind Community responding? What more could they possibly want?

Eventually, we had to face the facts. The Blind Community simply wasn't interested, for some reason, in our show. I threw my hands up and called the rest of the Gideon Team and the Sheen Center to let them know I was canceling the assistive listening devices for that performance. They all congratulated me for trying so hard and we all agreed to focus on the other two outreach initiatives.

I turned my attention to the Deaf Community. I had hired two of the best interpreters in New York, Dylan Geil and Lusanne Massaro, and we had a huge response to our email and phone call outreach.

The interpreters were going to reach out to their communities and one of my close friends is deeply engaged with the Deaf Community. But still, as we got closer, the tickets set aside for the Deaf Community hadn't sold. Not one. We had received rave reviews in publications all over the city, we were selling out every single performance and those audiences were raving. Why weren't deaf audiences coming to the show? Again I asked myself, what more could they possibly want? We couldn't cancel the performance, I'd already hired the interpreters and the show was already selling out with other audience members, but we ended up having only one deaf audience member – a friend of ours who bought his ticket a few hours before the show.

Three out of the four felt like total failures. I told myself that I had been magnanimous and generous but... maybe these communities simply weren't interested in our show. Maybe theatre itself is such a difficult sell that these people weren't going to come no matter what I did.

The performance for parents was turning into a bigger success. Because I have two kids of my own, my personal community is all theatre people and parents. A group of my theatre-parent friends had reserved tickets for the show and on the day, we had four teaching artists doing theatre games and building art projects with the kids while their parents watched the performance. It was the only successful bit of outreach we'd done.

The show closed and as part of the depression/ decompression that accompanies a closing show, I looked back on the outreach. I had written the whole thing off as a failed experiment. But the recurring question, "What more could they possibly want?" went from a comforting mantra to a nagging question that needed to be answered. The more times I asked myself that, the closer I came to an uncomfortable truth. We wanted to reach out to four different communities, but I was only personally invested in one of them. I have kids, I know a lot of people who have kids. We share stories, we have playdates. We set up a show for parents because parents came to us and said, "I wish you had a show for us." That's something they wanted.

When it comes to outreach, we have to be really careful about cultural appropriation. And that's essentially what I had done with the other three groups. I don't suffer from a disability that would keep me out of the theatre and I don't personally know anyone who is deaf or blind. In fact, I had to check with several people just to suss out the right language – are they hearing impaired or deaf? Visually impaired or blind? I had no idea.

As a counterpoint, some years ago we decided to change our hiring and casting practices to be more diverse and inclusive. This has been hugely successful for us – our audiences are more diverse and our shows are more vibrant and artistically informed. But the reason we did it is because we were asked to do it. A friend came up to me at the end of a show and said, "You don't know how frustrating it is to see a play this good with almost no people of color. I want you to do more, I want you to do better." And we've tried.

With the Disability Outreach, it was as if I walked up to the door of a community center that I had never been to before and said, "I have one single performance set aside for you, you're welcome. By the way, my name is Sean. See you at the theatre!" When I think back to how frustrated I was that the Blind Community didn't respond to my emails and letters without considering that written text might not be the best way to contact them, I feel considerable shame. The solution moving forward is to be in touch with these communities as we begin to plan our productions and actually ask them, "What more can we do? What more do you want?" and then see if there's a way to implement those suggestions.

We can't confuse outreach with investment. I was measuring the response to my initiatives in terms of audience members who showed up at the theatre, but that means I was looking to capitalize on an underserved community instead of legitimately serving them. As we look forward at 2017 and beyond, I intend to be in dialogue with these communities because that's the only way I will know what I have to do to make all of these people feel welcome at our productions.

GLOSSARY

This glossary is by no means inclusive of every term you will come across in your work in disability and inclusion theatre, there are numerous terms and new technologies being created and coined weekly. This is but a dip in the waters of the language you will use, the disabilities you will encounter and technology you will deal with and should be more than enough to lay out the basics and get you off on the right foot. Again, the internet is a great tool to search for any further terms, technologies, information about disabilities you do not understand, disability rights and advocates or general information.

Ableism   Discrimination in favor of able-bodied people. Using words such as 'retarded' can be called ableist slurs. People who discriminate are known as ableist.

Access-A-Ride   Access-A-Ride provides transportation for people with disabilities whose disability prevents their use of accessible mass transit, public bus or subway service for some or all of their trips. Access-A-Ride is operated by private carriers under contract to New York City. Similar ride providers exist in your community, search them out.

Activity-dependent plasticity   A form of functional and structural neuroplasticity that arises from the use of cognitive functions and personal experience; hence, it is the biological basis for learning and the formation of new memories. Activity-dependent plasticity is a form of neuroplasticity that arises from intrinsic or endogenous activity, as opposed to forms of neuroplasticity that arise from extrinsic or exogenous factors, such as electrical brain stimulation or drug-induced neuroplasticity. The brain's ability to remodel itself forms the basis of the brain's capacity to retain memories, improve motor function and enhance comprehension and speech amongst other things.

ADA The Americans with Disabilities Act (ADA) prohibits discrimination against people with disabilities in employment, transportation, public accommodation, communications and governmental activities.

ADA compliant Among other things, the ADA ensures access to the built environment for people with disabilities. The ADA Standards establish design requirements for the construction and alteration of facilities subject to the law. These enforceable standards apply to places of public accommodation, commercial facilities and state and local government facilities. Adherence to these standards make you ADA compliant.

ADHD Attention deficit hyperactivity disorder is a neuro-developmental disorder. It is characterized by problems paying attention, excessive activity or difficulty controlling behavior.

AEA Actors Equity Association. The union for stage actors in the US.

AFTRA Originally the American Federation of Television and Radio Artists. In 2012 it merged with Screen Actors Guild, the film union, and now is SAG-AFTRA.

Alopecia universalis A medical condition, thought to be autoimmune in nature, involving loss of all body hair, including eyebrows and eyelashes.

ASL American Sign Language is the primary sign language used by deaf and hearing-impaired people in the US and Canada, devised in part by Thomas Hopkins Gallaudet on the basis of sign language in France.

Assistive listening Any technology that enhances the understanding of speech by people with hearing impairments in acoustic environments in which speech is distorted, muffled or obscured by background noise.

Assistivetech.net The US national public website on assistive technology. Every theatre company should visit this site, as should every university.

Audio description An additional narration track intended primarily for blind and visually-impaired consumers of visual media (including television and film, dance, opera and visual art). Audio description is frequently done live during live theatre and music performances.

Autism and Autism spectrum disorder (ASD) are both general terms for a group of complex disorders of brain development. These disorders are characterized, in varying degrees, by difficulties in social interaction and verbal and non-verbal communication, and repetitive behaviors.

Basecamp Basecamp is a private, secure space online where people working together can organize and discuss everything they need to get a project done. See it, track it, discuss it, act on it. Tasks, discussions, deadlines and files – everything's predictably organized in Basecamp.

Braille A system of writing and printing for blind- or visually-impaired people, in which varied arrangements of raised dots representing letters and numerals are identified by touch.

BSL British Sign Language.

Cochlear implants A surgically implanted electronic device that provides a sense of sound to a person who is profoundly deaf or hard of hearing in both ears. Cochlear implants bypass the normal hearing process; they have a microphone and some electronics that reside outside the skin, generally behind the ear, which transmit a signal to an array of electrodes placed in the cochlea, which stimulate the cochlear nerve.

Co-playing A stage performance style where two actors, one deaf and one hearing, perform the same role simultaneously. The 'co' implies mutual ownership of the role.

CP Cerebral palsy is a disorder that affects muscle tone, movement and motor skills (the ability to move in a coordinated and purposeful way). It may affect five different people in five completely different ways.

Cross-disability casting The process of casting disabled actors in roles which are disabled, but do not have the same disability as the actor.

CSL Cyprus/Cypriot Sign Language.

DASL The Director of ASL coordinates the translation of a text into ASL, pins down the meanings and the issues the director wants to address, and offers correction or new word ideas to ASL signing actors or interpreters.

Deaf (deaf) It has become accepted that a capital 'D' refers to Deaf people as a culture. Lowercase 'd' deaf refers to deafness or hearing loss. Capital 'D' Deaf people identify themselves as culturally Deaf. Lowercase 'd' deaf people generally do not associate with culturally Deaf people.

Disability culture Behaviors, beliefs, ways of living that are unique to persons affected by disability. Three common ways of thinking about disability culture are (1) historical, (2) social and political and (3) personal and aesthetic, which emphasizes a way of living and positive identification with being disabled.

Disability theatre Disability theatre is all about ensuring disabled people are at the center of the creative process, and allowing disability to influence that process.

Drama therapy Drama therapy is the intentional use of drama and/or theatre processes to achieve therapeutic goals.

Epilepsy A group of neurological disorders marked by varying types and intensities of seizures.

Grab bars Bars attached to a wall to provide a grip, e.g., near a bathtub or next to a toilet, for people who have difficulty in standing up.

Grand mal seizures The most common and dramatic, and therefore the most well known, is the generalized convulsion, also called the grand mal seizure. In this type of seizure, the patient loses consciousness and usually collapses.

Helen Keller (June 27, 1880–June 1, 1968) was an American author, political activist, and lecturer. She was the first deaf-blind person to earn a Bachelor of Arts degree. The story of how Keller's teacher, Anne Sullivan, broke through the isolation imposed by a complete lack of language, allowing the girl to blossom as she learned to communicate, has become widely known through the dramatic depictions of the play and film *The Miracle Worker*.

HIV/AIDS Human immunodeficiency virus infection and acquired immune deficiency syndrome (HIV/AIDS) is a spectrum of conditions caused by infection with the human immunodeficiency virus.

Identity-first language (IFL) Mode of address adopted by most autistic, blind, deaf and some mobility-impaired people. It treats the condition (i.e., autistic man) as part of the identity of the person and therefore of great value.

Inclusion The action or state of including or of being included within a group or structure.

Inspiration porn Inspiration porn is an image of a person with a disability, often a kid, doing something completely ordinary – like playing, or talking, or running, or drawing a picture, or hitting a tennis ball – carrying a caption like 'Your excuse is invalid' or 'Before you quit, try'. Using these images as feel-good tools, as 'inspiration,' is based on an assumption that the people in them have terrible lives, and that it takes some extra kind of pluck or courage to live them.

Intersectionality A term used to describe the overlapping of social identities (age, race, disability) in one person, population, project or group and the related societal systems of oppression or discrimination.

Intimacy of disability A term referring to the circle of intimacy a director or choreographer is trusted enough to be drawn into with a disabled performer.

LGBTQIA Well-known acronym meaning lesbian, gay, bisexual, transgendered and questioning. Additionally there is occasionally an I added before or after the Q to signify intersex and a newer addition of an A for asexual, agender, aromantic.

Mainstreaming Integration of children with special educational problems, as a physical handicap, into conventional classes and school activities but in separate disabled groups.

MS Multiple sclerosis is a disease in which the insulating covers of nerve cells in the brain and spinal cord are damaged. This damage disrupts the ability of parts of the nervous system to communicate, resulting in a range of signs and symptoms, including physical, mental and sometimes psychiatric problems.

NEA The National Endowment for the Arts is an independent federal agency that funds, promotes and strengthens the creative capacity of our communities by providing all Americans with diverse opportunities for arts participation.

Neurodiversity/neurotypical Terms referring either to the variation in anatomy, functions and organic disorders of nerves and the nervous system or to the 'normative' state of such. This is a new way to address neurological states, injuries, stages and ways of being without an academic or medical slant that may be prejudicial.

Neuroplasticity Also known as brain plasticity or neural plasticity, neuroplasticity is an umbrella term that describes lasting change to the brain throughout an individual's life course. The term gained prominence in the latter half of the twentieth century, when new research showed that many aspects of the brain can be altered (or are 'plastic') even into adulthood. This notion is in contrast with the previous scientific consensus that the brain develops during a critical period in early childhood and then remains relatively unchanged (or 'static').

NYITA, The New York Innovative Theatre Award The New York Innovative Theatre Foundation was created to bring recognition to the great work being done in New York City's Off-Off-Broadway community, to honor its artistic heritage, and to provide a meeting ground for this extensive community. Once a year it honors its finest with the NYITAs.

OCD Obsessive-compulsive disorder is a mental disorder where people feel the need to check things repeatedly, perform certain routines repeatedly (called 'rituals') or have certain thoughts repeatedly. People usually are unable to control either the thoughts or the activities for more than a short period of time.

People-first language (PFL) Linguistics which place an individual before their handicap by depicting what an individual has rather than equating the person with the handicap. This has traditionally been used by social services, government or education bodies. Also known as person-first language.

Petit mal seizure Also called absence seizures. They cause a short loss of consciousness (just a few seconds) with few or no symptoms. The patient, most often a child, typically interrupts an activity and stares blankly.

Polio   Polio is a contagious viral illness that in its most severe form causes paralysis, difficulty breathing and sometimes death. In the US, the last case of naturally occurring polio happened in 1979.

PWD   Person with a disability. In this usage I am referring to the American acting unions' movement involving artists with disabilities working in the arts, not any of the international PWD movements or activities.

PTSD   Post-traumatic stress disorder. Stress-related symptoms from traumatic events which may include mood swings, flashbacks or uncontrollable emotions. Not enough study has been done on PTSD in people with both physical and mental disabilities, however it does exist. Moreover, from children on up, those with disabilities suffering with PTSD can be helped.

SAG   Screen Actors Guild. The American union for film actors, which in 2012 merged with American Federation of Television and Radio Artists (AFTRA), becoming SAG-AFTRA.

SE   Signed English is a sign language dialect which matches each spoken word of English. It is mostly used for language development, allowing a teacher to reinforce the spoken word with its equivalent sign.

SEE   Signed Exact English is a signed language system that represents literal English. It is a tool to make visible everything that is not heard.

Sensory friendly   Adaptations to, or staging of, a performance which makes it a performing arts experience that is welcoming to all families with children with autism or with other disabilities that create sensory sensitivities. Some aspects include: lower sound levels; elimination of potentially startling special effects and lighting; house lights on at about twenty percent; relaxed house rules – you are free to get up, move around, and leave if needed; allowed use of iPads and other electronics for therapeutic uses; volunteers scattered throughout the theatre to assist and direct audience members as needed; quiet areas and activity areas in the lobby for taking a break; and trained staff, ushers and volunteers.

Social Stories   Social Stories are short descriptive pieces of text, which use images to describe to the child with autism the skill or situation – like a comic script conversation. Always written in first person text and from the child's own point of view. The social skills story will answer the ever important 'wh' questions – who, what, where, when and why as well as 'How' and provide an insight into the thoughts, feelings and emotions of others which is an area of marked weakness for most children with ASD. Phamaly Theatre provides the most comprehensive use of Social Stories to date.

TAB A slang term used in the disability community to mean 'temporarily able bodied' when referring to a non-disabled person.

Tactile or 'touch' tours Tours of the set given to audience members who have visual disabilities. These tours take place before the show where the audience member may be allowed to walk on and touch the set and various props. They may also have a particularly important set piece explained to them. The set is then oriented in space for them before the show begins.

TBI Traumatic brain injury, also known as intracranial injury, occurs when an external force traumatically injures the brain. TBI can be classified based on severity, mechanism, or other features. Head injury usually refers to TBI, but is a broader category because it can involve damage to structures other than the brain, such as the scalp and skull.

TTY/TDD TTY/TDD stands for a group of telecommunication devices that make it easier for deaf and/or mute people to talk over telephone lines. TTY stands for telephone typewriter, teletypewriter or text phone. TDD stands for telecommunications device for the deaf.

UFAS Uniform Federal Accessibility Standards. They set standards for facility accessibility by physically handicapped persons for Federal and federally-funded facilities. These standards are to be applied during the design, construction and alteration of buildings and facilities to the extent required by the Architectural Barriers Act of 1968, as amended.

VIA Visually Impaired Apps is an app from the Braille Institute which has been designed to help identify apps that are useful for adults and children who are blind or visually impaired. These apps generally verbalize directions or can vocalize dialogue programming into them, such as lines of a text or book.

Vibratory cues   Any cue used in staging which is vibratory in nature. This can include banging, music, throwing an object, foot stomping, gently knocking and more. Imagination is the key.

Wee-wee pads   A pad of absorbent cotton for the dog to urinate on if it cannot go outside.

WheelMate   WheelMate™ is a global environmental accessibility mapping program for people with mobility disabilities, walking disabilities and other disabilities that require that the indoor or outdoor environment be adapted to be completely accessible. It is helpful for finding wheelchair-accessible toilets and parking spaces. (www.wheelmate.com Accessed 27 February 2017. Also available as a smartphone app.)

BIBLIOGRAPHY AND RESOURCES

This is not an exhaustive list by any means and you should dip into the world of plays, authors, life stories and classics in disability studies. This list is enough to get you started.

Print and online bibliography

Barnett, Sharon N. 'Disability Culture or Disability Consciousness' (Abstract). *Journal of Disability Policy Studies*. Summer 1996 vol. 7 no. 2 1–19. http://dps.sagepub.com/content/7/2/1.abstract accessed 27 February 2017.

Barton-Farcas, Stephanie. 'Against Sameness in Theatre.' HowlRound. Emerson College. October 28, 2015. http://howlround.com/against-sameness-in-theatre accessed 27 February 2017.

Belluso, John. *Henry Flamethrowa, Pyretown, A Nervous Smile, The Rules of Charity.* New York: Dramatists Play Service (separate scripts), 2006–2008.

Belluso, John. *Gretty Good Time, Sleeping City, Traveling Skin.* New York: Playscripts (separate scripts), 2005–2009.

Brenna, Beverley A. *Stories for Every Classroom: Canadian Fiction Portraying Characters with Disabilities.* Toronto, Canada: Canadian Scholars Press, May 2015.

Browning, Tim. '1984.' *Theaterscene.net.* April 16, 2003. http://spoontheater.org/reviews/Theaterscene.pdf

Carlson, Tiffany. *10 Things the World can Learn from People with Disabilities.* The Mobility Resource Blog. https://blog.themobilityresource.com/blog/post/10-things-the-world-can-learn-from-people-with-disabilities/ accessed 27 February 2017.

Cino, Maggie. 'Innovative Double Casting'. *United Stages.* 2005. http://spoontheater.org/reviews/us05.pdf

Clare, Eli. *Brilliant Imperfection: Grappling with Cure.* Durham, NC: Duke University Press Books, 2017.

Davidson, Michael. *Concerto for the Left Hand: Disability and the Defamiliar Body.* Michigan, MI: University of Michigan Press, 2008.

Davis, Lennard J., ed. *The Disability Studies Reader.* New York: Routledge, 1997.

DiDonato, Tiffanie. *Dwarf: A Memoir.* New York: Plume, 2012.

Dunn, Katherine. *Geek Love.* New York: Alfred A. Knopf, 1989.

Elias-Reyes, Rohana. 'Sleeping Handsome.' *Nytheatre.com* (Now a legacy site of Nytheater Indie Archive and soon to be live online) 2008.

Garland-Thomson, Rosemarie. *Extraordinary Bodies: Figuring Physical Disability in American Culture and Literature.* New York: Columbia University Press, 1997.

Greenwald, Laurie. *Thank You.* Private Letter To Nicu's Spoon Company. 2007.

Haddon, Mark. *The Curious Incident of the Dog in the Nighttime.* New York: Doubleday, 2003.

Inclusion in the Arts. 'The Language of Disability: Do's and Don'ts' http://inclusioninthearts.org/faqs/the-language-of-disability-dos-and-donts/ accessed 8 March 2017.

Johnston, Kirsty. *Disability Theatre and Modern Drama: Recasting Modernism.* New York: Methuen, 2016.

Krivohlavek, Amy. 'A Theater of Diversity: Nicu's Spoon Launches New Season With Lost Formicans'. *OffOffOnline.* March 28, 2007. www.offoffonline.com/offoffonline/392?rq=amy%20krivohlavek

Kuusisto, Stephen. *Planet of the Blind.* New York: Delta Press, 1998.

Lewis, Victoria Ann, ed. *Beyond Victims and Villains: Contemporary Plays by Disabled Playwrights.* New York: Theatre Communications Group, 2006.

Linton, Simi. *My Body Politic.* Ann Arbor, MI: University of Michigan Press, 2006.

Linton, Simi. *Claiming Disability: Knowledge & Identity.* New York: NYU Press, 1998.

Livingston, Donovan. *Lift Off: Harvard Graduation Speech.* 2016. www.youtube.com/watch?v=9xgupkitejm

Moore, John. 'Summer Arts Guide, Theater.' *The Denver Post*. June 1, 2006. www.denverpost.com/2006/06/01/summer-arts-guide-theater/

Palacios, Maria R. *Criptionary: Disability Humor and Satire*. New York: Atahualpa Press, 2013.

Rothbart, Brad. 'Once More Unto the Breach: An Anatomized Philippic Regarding the Relationship of Disability to the Contemporary American Theatre.' *American Theatre Magazine*, November 2015. http://www.americantheatre.org/2015/10/20/once-more-unto-the-breach/ accessed 27 February 2017.

Russell, Marta. *Beyond Ramps: Disability at the End of the Social Contract*. Monroe, ME: Common Courage Press, 2002.

Russell, Ron. 'Bent Voices.' *San Francisco Observer*. 2005. www.bentvoices.org/bentvoices/belluso_memorial.htm

Shakespeare Teacher. 'Theatre: *Richard III* At Nicu's Spoon.' July 22, 2007. www.shakespeareteacher.com/blog/archives/277

Solomon, Andrew. *Far From The Tree*. New York: Scribner, 2012.

Tammett, Daniel. *Born on A Blue Day: Inside the Extraordinary Mind of an Autistic Savant*. New York: Free Press, 2007.

Titchkosky, Tanya. *The Question of Access: Disability, Space, Meaning*. Toronto, Canada: University of Toronto Press, 2011.

Two And Twenty Troubles. Directed By Victor Ilyukhin. 2015. SVA, New York. www.22troublesfilm.com/

Viagas, Robert. 'Off-Off-Broadway Company Plans Richard III With All Differently Abled Actors.' *Playbill*. September 1, 2015. www.playbill.com/article/off-off-broadway-company-plans-richard-iii-with-all-differently-abled-actors-com-360471

Wright, David. *Deafness: A Personal Account*. London: Allen Lane, 1969.

Websites as Resources

http://routledge.com/cw/barton-farcas   Companion website to this book which includes thirty different worksheets, guides and checklists for use in theaters and universities.

http://inclusioninthearts.org   The Alliance for Inclusion in the Arts is the US's leading advocate for full diversity as a key to the vitality and dynamism of American theatre, film and television. They promote authentic dialogue about race, culture and disability that embraces the complexity of underlying social and historical issues. accessed 27 February 2017.

www.disabilityartsinternational.org/ Disability Arts International is a British website that promotes increased access to the arts for disabled artists and audiences around the globe. They have a new directory which any and all groups working in inclusive and disability theatre should be on. accessed 27 February 2017.

http://aplusa.org/ The adaptation + ability group is a technical and social laboratory for creative research on technology and the body at Olin College, Needham, MA. They are interested in the encounters between humans and the built environment – especially when there's a mismatch between standardized design and the atypical body or mind. But they are also interested in critical questions about the future of the body: What counts as normal? accessed 27 February 2017.

https://smartasscripple.blogspot.com Mike Ervin's Blog. Expressing pain through sarcasm since 2010. Welcome to the official site for bitter cripples (and those who love them). Smart Ass Cripple has been voted World's Biggest Smart Ass by J.D. Power and Associates. accessed 27 February 2017.

http://www.22troublesfilm.com/ *Two and Twenty Troubles* website. Documentary about Nicu's Spoon Theater Company and the artists who work in it and in New York City. accessed 27 February 2017.

http://dragaleg.blogspot.com/ Blog of Mallory Kay Nelson, a designer who works with and for disabled artists. She is a Disability Designer Specialist taking on Hollywood and the film and television and theatre industry as we know it! accessed 27 February 2017.

http://askjan.org/bulletins/adaaa1.htm The Job Accommodation Network (JAN) is the leading source of free, expert and confidential guidance on workplace accommodations and disability employment issues. Working toward practical solutions that benefit both employer and employee, JAN helps people with disabilities enhance their employability, and shows employers how to capitalize on the value and talent that people with disabilities add to the workplace. accessed 27 February 2017.

https://disabledperson.com a premier Job Board for People with Disabilities since 2002. They boast over 250,000 active USA jobs with hundreds and even thousands of new jobs posted every day. Jobs are posted by companies who are looking to hire people with disabilities. The pages on disabledperson.com can act like maps to guide you to your future job. accessed 27 February 2017.

http://disabilitycinemacoalition.weebly.com/ The Disability Cinema Coalition (DCC) is a network of organizations dedicated to the empowerment and inclusion of people with disabilities within the cinematic arts. accessed 27 February 2017.

www.semel.ucla.edu/nadc The National Arts and Disability Center (NADC) promotes the full inclusion of audiences and artists with disabilities into all facets of the arts community. The NADC is a leading consultant in the arts and disability community, and the only center of its kind. The information is aimed at artists with disabilities, arts organizations, arts administrators, disability organizations, performing arts organizations, art centers, universities and arts educators. accessed 27 February 2017.

www.ableize.com/ ABLEize is the largest and most viewed UK disability resource offering the largest collection of disability, mobility and health websites and social media pages in the UK and Europe. ABLEize was born out of the frustration of its founder, a disabled wheelchair user, following poor internet search results and is now the most comprehensive directory of disability and health care information and products on the internet. ABLEize promotes quality, trusted information, advice, products and services as well as education, disabled support groups, local clubs and sports and much more. It is also the ideal platform to promote mobility, daily living aids and disability shopping sites. It is a fabulous international reference point with theatre and arts groups, travel recommendations, education, products and much more. accessed 27 February 2017.

http://disartfestival.org/ DisArt aims to change perceptions about disability, one work of art at a time. They believe that the creative act can stimulate important, necessary civic conversation and influence cultural change. By celebrating art practices that aim to elevate an understanding of the human condition of disability, they encourage all people, disabled or not, to appreciate the complex identities of those around them. By increasing access to exemplary examples of disability art and culture, DisArt awakens a spirit of ability, equality, social inclusion, physical accessibility, community and a sense of place for those living with disability. accessed 27 February 2017.

www.ada.gov/websites2.htm Accessibility of State and Local Government Websites to People with Disabilities: the Internet is dramatically changing the way that American government serves the public. Taking advantage of new technology, many State and local governments are using the web to offer citizens a host of services spotlighted on this site. accessed 27 February 2017.

Associations and Inclusive Theatre Companies in the US

Adaptive Arts Theater, New York: www.adaptiveartstheater.org accessed 27 February 2017.

The Apothetae, New York: www.theapothetae.org accessed 27 February 2017.

Asperger's Are Us, Boston, MA: www.facebook.com/aspergersareus accessed 27 February 2017.

Bodies of Work: A Network of Disability Art and Culture, Chicago, IL: http://ahs.uic.edu/disability-human-development/community-partners/bodies-of-work/ accessed 12 March 2017.

Deaf West Theatre, Los Angeles, CA: www.deafwest.org accessed 27 February 2017.

Dionysus Theatre Company, Houston, TX: www.dionysustheatre.net accessed 27 February 2017.

First Stage Theater, Milwaukee, WI: www.firststage.org accessed 27 February 2017.

Gideon Productions, New York: www.gideonth.com accessed 27 February 2017.

Mixed Blood Theatre Company, Minneapolis, MN: www.mixedblood.com accessed 27 February 2017.

National Theatre of the Deaf, New London, CT: www.ntd.org accessed 27 February 2017.

New York Deaf Theatre, Brooklyn, NY: www.newyorkdeaftheatre.org/ accessed 27 February 2017.

Nicu's Spoon Theater Company, New York: www.spoontheater.org accessed 27 February 2017.

Phamaly Theatre Company, Denver, CO: www.phamaly.org accessed 27 February 2017.

Sins Invalid, San Francisco, CA: www.sinsinvalid.org accessed 27 February 2017.

TBTB (Theater Breaking Through Barriers), New York: www.tbtb. org accessed 27 February 2017.

Tellin' Tales Theatre Company, Chicago, IL: www.tellintales.org accessed 27 February 2017.

That Uppity Theatre Company, Saint Louis, MO: www.uppityco. com accessed 27 February 2017.

Associations and Groups outside the US

Australia

Back to Back Theatre: http://backtobacktheatre.com accessed 27 February 2017.

No Strings Attached Theatre of Disability: www.nostringsattached. org.au

Options Theatre Company: www.facebook.com/Options-Theatre-Company-339500652793232 accessed 27 February 2017.

Canada

Workman Arts: www.workmanarts.com accessed 27 February 2017.

Germany

Theater Sycorax: www.theatersycorax.de/1/theater-sycorax accessed 27 February 2017.

Japan

Performance Troupe TAIHEN: www.ne.jp/asahi/imaju/taihen accessed 27 February 2017.

The Netherlands

Theater Maatwerk: www.theatermaatwerk.nl/en accessed 27 February 2017.

Sweden

Moomsteatern: http://moomsteatern.com accessed 27 February 2017.

Switzerland

Theater HORA: www.hora.ch/2013/index.php?s=2 accessed 27 February 2017.

UK

Birds of Paradise Theatre Company: www.boptheatre.co.uk accessed 27 February 2017.

Face Front Inclusive Theatre: http://facefront.org accessed 27 February 2017.

The Freewheelers Theatre and Media Company: www. freewheelerstheatre.co.uk accessed 27 February 2017.

Graeae Theatre Company: http://graeae.org accessed 27 February 2017.

TwoCan Inclusive Theatre Company: www.twocantheatre.org.uk accessed 27 February 2017.

INDEX

Note: Page numbers in *italic* refer to illustrations.

Printed in Great Britain
by Amazon